SOLVING PATIENT PROBLEMS:

Psychiatry

SOLVING PATIENT PROBLEMS:

Psychiatry

Terry A. Travis, M.D., M.S.Ed.

Professor Emeritus of Psychiatry
and Medical Education
Southern Illinois University School
of Medicine
Staff Psychiatrist
Memorial Medical Center
St. John's Hospital
Springfield, Illinois

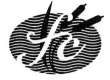

Typesetter: Pagesetters, Brattleboro, VT
Printer: Port City Press, Baltimore, MD

Distributors:

United States and Canada
Blackwell Science, Inc.
Commerce Place
350 Main Street
Malden, MA 02148
Telephone orders: 800-215-1000 or 781-388-8250
Fax orders: 781-388-8270

Australia
Blackwell Science, PTY LTD.
54 University Street
Carlton, Victoria 3053
Telephone orders: 61-39-347-0300
Fax orders: 61-39-347-5001

Outside North America and Australia
Blackwell Science, LTD.
c/o Marston Book Service, LTD.
P.O. Box 269
Abingdon Oxon, OX 14 4XN England
Telephone orders: 44-1-235-465500

2 3 4 5 6 7 8 9 10

Contents

Contributors

David H. Decker, M.D.
Associate Professor
Department of Psychiatry
Southern Illinois University School of Medicine
Medical Director
Adolescent Center
Memorial Medical Center
Springfield, Illinois

Ronald W. Kanwischer, M.A., C.A.D.C.
Assistant Professor
Department of Psychiatry
Southern Illinois University School of Medicine
Addiction Program Director
Memorial Medical Center
Springfield, Illinois

Robert J. Pary, M.D.
Associate Professor
Department of Psychiatry
Southern Illinois University School of Medicine
Springfield, Illinois
Clinical Director
Lincoln Developmental Center
Lincoln, Illinois

Preface

This book provides a clinical approach for primary physicians for the initial diagnosis and treatment of psychiatric disorders. The structure of this text is based on the clinical reasoning process, and the outlines of each chapter represent the thought process followed when evaluating a patient. This guide also suggests when referral to a psychiatrist is indicated.

Emphasis is placed on the diagnostic process and on the initial treatment of patients with uncomplicated and clearly diagnosed psychiatric illnesses. Taking a thorough history and performing a complete mental status examination are emphasized. General treatment guidelines are used, as most patients have a straightforward diagnosis and respond well to the usual treatment. Patients who are not easily diagnosed or who do not respond to or have significant problems with the usual treatment should be referred to a psychiatrist. This book was written to be a quick resource that clarifies the thought process behind the diagnosis, reminds the physician of the differential diagnosis, and provides initial treatment recommendations for the patient.

Each chapter is divided into several sections that represent the clinical approach to the patient. The *definition* provides a brief explanation of each category of mental illness. The *chief complaint* section provides examples of typical complaints of patients with these illnesses. The section on the *differential diagnosis* includes a list of medical illnesses that must be ruled out prior to making the psychiatric diagnosis, as well as suggestions for screening procedures and laboratory tests that should be performed prior to initiating treatment. This section also contains algorithms that review the diagnostic process for these specific psychiatric diagnoses. This is followed by a section that presents the *specific disorder*, including a description of the criteria from the *Diagnostic and Statistical Manual of Mental Disorders*, 4th ed. *(DSM-IV)*. Clinical questions and clinical observations are provided. Clinical questions are suggestions to be used during the interview to clarify and detail the patient's history and specific symptoms. They are a how-to guide for face-to-face interaction with the patient. The clinical observations provide a guide to the mental status observations made by the physician while working with the patient. Brief cases are provided to illustrate the specific psychiatric disorder under discussion. Another section provides an overview of *treatment* approaches, and a final section summarizes the *epidemiological* or other clinically useful information.

The logic of this text should aid and simplify the physician's approach to the patient who presents with a psychiatric complaint. It should also help to rule out medical illnesses and to establish an accurate psychiatric diagnosis on which to base treatment recommendations or a decision to refer.

TERRY A. TRAVIS, M.D., M.S.ED.

This book is dedicated to the many patients and students with whom I have worked over the past 30 years.

Introduction

One of the major problems in medical education is that the traditional approach (memory-based approach) to educating future physicians inadequately prepares them for solving patient problems. Thus, problem-based learning was designed to place the teaching of content (and memorization) and problem-solving skills on an equal footing. Surveys of both traditional and problem-based educational programs have determined the following: most students in traditional programs feel that more than 50% of what they learn is memorized without understanding; however, most students in problem-based programs feel that less than 20% of what they learn is memorized without understanding. Unfortunately, because of the deficiencies in the traditional (memory-based) approach to medicine, students are handicapped by their memorization of large amounts of information that they are unable to apply to clinical problems.

These books are designed to help the reader develop an approach to clinical problem-solving. While traditional medical education demands that students memorize vast amounts of information without understanding, problem-based learning is based on the concept of practicing the process of problem-solving while acquiring the knowledge (content) used in the process. George Bordage, M.D.,[1] states in his article "Elaborated Knowledge" that "less is better for beginning students when introducing new material"; that is, in order for the student to be able to organize information for later recall, less information, preferably using prototypical case presentations, must be provided so that students are able to understand, incorporate, and then use what they learn. Students who have the most trouble with clinical reasoning seem to have a poorly organized knowledge base, making rational approaches to patient problems almost impossible.

There is no question that knowledge is important in problem-solving. The more the student knows, the better he or she can test the hypotheses that are entertained. It is the quality of the hypotheses and the skill in testing them that distinguish the expert from the novice. Failure to consider more than one hypotheses is one of

[1] Bordage G: Elaborated knowledge: a key to successful diagnostic thinking. *Acad Med* 69:883-885, 1994. George Bordage, M.D., is Professor and Director of Graduate Studies in the Department of Medical Education at the College of Medicine, University of Illinois at Chicago, Chicago, Illinois.

the basic deficiencies of inexperience. One of the goals of this text is to help the student move from novice to expert in this critical area of medical diagnosis.

The purpose of the *Solving Patient Problems Series* is to assist students at all levels in developing their clinical problem-solving or reasoning skills by leading them through the "clinical reasoning process around common presenting complaints" in the various clinical rotations. The most common diseases that students are likely to encounter given the presenting complaints are presented. These prototypical diseases are the foundation upon which students may then begin to build a more extensive differential. Only by comparing and contrasting the diagnostic features of two or more common diseases can students build a knowledge base that will allow the inclusion of other possible causes of the same complaint, thereby moving from prototypical problems to more complex problems and then to life-threatening problems that must not be overlooked.

In no way is this text meant to be inclusive but rather a supplement, guide, and aid to the success of students as diagnosticians. It is deliberately pocket-sized to be carried on clinical rotations. More extensive reading about patients is necessary. However, facts learned about diseases in the context of patient presentations are bound to be easier to retain and retrieve. What seems to be "intuition" and part of the "art" of medicine is actually a combination of experience and a very highly organized knowledge base, which allows physicians to differentiate quickly between differential diagnoses—a necessary skill that this text has been designed to help students develop.

S. SCOTT OBENSHAIN, M.D.[2]

---

[2] S. Scott Obenshain, M.D., is the Associate Dean for Undergraduate Medical Education and Professor of Pediatrics and Family and Community Medicine at the University of New Mexico School of Medicine, Albuquerque, New Mexico.

CHAPTER 1
Psychiatry:
Definition and Overview

Terry A. Travis, M.D., M.S.Ed.

DEFINITION

Psychiatry is the medical specialty that assesses, diagnoses, and treats mental disorders. Mental disorders and diseases are defined by the patient's pattern of disturbed thought, emotions, and behavior. Psychiatrists treat diseases of the part of the brain that performs the higher mental processes involved with the interpretation of stimuli, feelings resulting from that interpretation, and, ultimately, the behavioral response to the stimulus. This high-level cognitive and integrative mental process makes each of us unique. In contrast, the field of neurology is concerned with the more primitive areas of the brain that maintain the vital motor and sensory functions.

This book approaches mental disorders from the perspective of the *medical model* of psychiatry. The assessment, diagnosis, and treatment of the mental disorder or illness requires the same clinical reasoning process a clinician uses to assess, diagnose, and treat a disorder or illness in any other part of the body. The medical model uses the scientific method to diagnose an illness reliably. The illness is then treated with a variety of therapies based on the scientific evidence of treatment efficacy.

OVERVIEW

Psychiatric diagnoses are based on clinical criteria that are determined by assessing and determining syndromes or patterns of signs, symptoms, and the course of the disorder. Mental disorders are classed or grouped on the basis of shared characteristics.

The *Diagnostic and Statistical Manual of Mental Disorders*, 4th ed. (*DSM-IV*), published by the American Psychiatric Association, is the currently accepted standard for the diagnosis of psychiatric disorders. It is descriptive in its approach and based on clinical features, and it systematically specifies diagnostic criteria for each mental disorder. The *DSM-IV* also evaluates the patient on five variables or axes.

Five Axes

Axis I covers all mental disorders except for those on Axis II. Axis I mental disorders include:

- Disorders of infancy, childhood, or adolescence
- Cognitive disorders, including delirium and dementia
- Substance-related disorders
- Schizophrenia and other psychotic disorders
- Mood disorders
- Anxiety disorders
- Somatoform, factitious, and dissociative disorders
- Adjustment disorders
- Personality disorders

Axis II covers developmental disorders and personality disorders.

Axis III is used to diagnose physical disorders or illnesses.

Axis IV covers psychosocial stressors of any kind, including:

- Problems with the primary support group
- Problems related to the social environment
- Educational problems
- Occupational problems
- Housing problems
- Economic problems
- Legal problems

Axis V is the global assessment of functioning (GAF) scale. The GAF scale ranges from 1–100.

- **0–40:** Psychosis is present and function is significantly impaired. Impairment ranges from representing a danger to oneself or others to not functioning in many areas of life.
- **40–70:** Both symptoms of a mental illness are present, and functioning is impaired. The physician should assign the lowest score possible based on either the severity of symptoms or impairment. The severity of symptoms and the degree of impairment typically (but not always) coincide. For example, a patient has serious symptoms of depression but has managed to continue functioning at work and socially. He or she would have a GAF score in the low 40s as a result of the symptoms of the illness. In contrast, a patient with minimal symptoms of depression who has stopped working and is not functioning on a day-to-day basis would also have a GAF score in the low 40s because of the severity of impaired function.
- **40–50:** Serious symptoms or impairment of function are present.
- **50–60:** Moderate symptoms or impairment of function are present.

- **60–70:** Mild symptoms or impairment of function are present.
- **70–90:** Minimal symptoms are present, and there is little or no impairment of function.
- **90–100:** No symptoms are present, and the patient exhibits superior function.

CHAPTER 2
Mental Status Examination

Terry A. Travis, M.D., M.S.Ed.

The mental status examination is an important and necessary part of every patient's evaluation. This portion of the patient's evaluation begins with the first contact, continues during the history taking, and finishes with a more formal, detailed inquiry into the patient's mental functioning. The mental status is the physical examination and review of systems of the portion of the brain that supports higher mental functions. Since the brain cannot be directly percussed or palpated, the mental status examination consists of two separate parts, observations and specific questions.

1. **Observations.** Begin evaluating the mental status by observing and listening to the patient. Many aspects of the patient's mental function can be noted by observation. The formal outline of the mental status provides a structure to record and review, ensuring that nothing is excluded.
2. **Specific Questions.** Directly question the patient to evaluate specific mental functions. To ask effective and comprehensive questions, the physician must practice repeatedly until he or she gets a feel for the usual and normal range of responses. Practice helps to bring questions to mind spontaneously and develops flexibility in using the mental status examination. This part of the examination takes 5–30 minutes.

The mental status examination is part of the history obtained from each patient and should be used as a basic format in write-ups and case presentations. The mental status should be placed in the patient's history between the review of systems (ROS) and the physical examination (PE). The patient's behavior and attitudes are described under the following headings:

- General behavior
- Speech
- Emotional state
- Thought processes
- Sensorium and mental capacity
- Insight and judgment

The mental status examination is outlined below.

MENTAL STATUS EXAMINATION OUTLINE

I.   **General Appearance, Attitude, and Behavior**

A. **Age and Grooming:** tidy, slovenly, neat, careless, dirty, decorative, mourning, immaculate, flamboyant

B. **Posture:** positions, restlessness, obvious tension

C. **Facial Expression:** smiling, crying, blank, scared, sad

D. **Manner and Attitude:** cooperative, resistant, sociable, reserved, reclusive, belligerent, negative, suspicious, apathetic, fearful, confident, overconfident, sarcastic, superior

E. **Psychomotor Activity:** hyperactive, hypoactive, bizarre gestures, mannerisms, posture, tics, gait, paralysis, tremors

II. **Speech:** volume, rate, latency, pushed or pressured, loquacious, retarded, mute, increased, decreased

III. **Emotional State (Mood and Affect):** elated, euphoric, calm, placid, depressed, perplexed, anxious, apathetic, flattened, labile, appropriate or inappropriate to situation

IV. **Thought Processes**

A. **Thought Form:** logical, coherent, circumstantial, loose associations, flight of ideas, clang associations, loss of goal

B. **Thought Content:** preoccupations, areas of concern, delusions, illusions, hallucinations, anxieties, phobia, compulsions, obsessions

V.   **Sensorium and Mental Capacity**

A. **Orientation:** place, time, person, and situation

B. **Memory**

1. **Recall of Remote Past Experience:** dates of education, military service, marriage, jobs

2. **Recall of Recent Past Experiences:** account of past 24 hours

3. **Recall of Immediate Impressions:** numbers, name objects, count digits forward and backward; repeat three words after 3 minutes

C. **Attention and Concentration:** digit repetitions, subtraction of serial sevens

D. **General Intellectual Evaluation:** name four presidents, governor, wars, recent newspaper reports, calculation, symbolization, proverb interpretation

VI. **Insight and Judgment:** realization and recognition of degree and nature of illness and current life circumstances; ability to make reasonable and practical plans; goals and ethics

MENTAL STATUS EXAMINATION

I. **General Appearance, Behavior, and Attitude.** This is a brief, vivid description of the patient. A colleague, after reading the description, should be able to recognize the patient by sight. It should include the following:

    A. **Age and Grooming.** Briefly describe the patient's dress, neatness, and the appropriateness of his or her appearance; list his or her apparent and real age.

    B. **Posture.** Posture includes the way the patient sits or lies during the interview, restlessness, tension, and bizarre or unusual positions.

    C. **Facial Expressions.** Briefly describe the appropriateness, mobility, and expression of emotion that are observed on the patient's face, such as alert, dull, stuporous, fearful, depressed, and elated.

    D. **Manner and Attitude.** Describe the patient's general manner and attitude during the interview. What impression does the patient make? Is he or she frightened, distracted, or angry?

    E. **Psychomotor Activity.** Describe in detail the motor activity observed. Is this activity increased or reduced? Are the patient's actions spontaneous? Does he or she initiate activity? Take note of the appropriateness of motor activity and of such things as compulsive rituals, fumbling with the bed clothes, assaultiveness, negative attitude, and attempts to escape. Is the patient restless, agitated, slowed, pacing, immobile, or tremulous? Are tics present?

II. **Speech.** The patient's style of talking should be studied carefully. Its various features should be recorded under the general headings of rate, form, and quantity. Is the speech slowed or accelerated? The quality of talk should also be noted, such as hesitating, whispering, shyness, humor, screaming, and mumbling. Is there a latent response? Is the speech pushed or pressured? Can the patient stop talking, when asked to do so?

III. **Emotional State.** The patient's emotional state should be evaluated in conjunction with the other examination findings and the history. This is essential to detect emotions that are not expressed verbally but are revealed by tone of voice, speech, and posture. A statement concerning the probable dependability of the patient's description should be included. The points to be stated in every record are:

A. **Mood.** Mood describes the general emotional state from the patient's *subjective* point of view and involves feelings that are present at the time of the examination and a few hours or days preceding it. It is best assessed by asking the patient directly and recording the response verbatim. Mood tends to be stable over time. Examples of descriptors are neutral, depressed, sad, angry, anxious, happy, and frightened.

B. **Affect.** Affect is the physician's *objective* assessment of the immediate emotional expression the patient reveals throughout the interview. A person may have a primarily depressed mood for several months but may have a brightened affect when talking about his or her children or job. The physician's duty as an interviewer is to attempt to elicit a full range of affect. Facets of affect to note include:

1. **Qualitative Descriptions.** Describe the type and intensity of emotions, whether of broad range or primarily evident with definite topics. Attention is focused on the emotions of depression, elation, euphoria, anger, anxiety, fear, suspiciousness, resentment, the absence of clearly experienced emotions or apathy, and emotional lability.

2. **Range.** Does the patient exhibit a full range of emotion (objectively) in response to the interview? Is the range constricted, blunted, or completely absent (flat)?

3. **Lability.** Are the patient's emotional reactions labile (quickly changing or unstable), or is he or she phlegmatic and not easily moved? Note the somatic evidence of emotions such as flushing, tachycardia, perspiration, tears, facial expression, and moist palms.

4. **Appropriateness to Content and Situation.** Is the patient's affect compatible and appropriate to the ideas being expressed, the general content of thought, and with his or her appearance and motor activity? Is it consistent with the patient's subjectively described mood? Is the patient's affect *not* compatible with these aspects of his or her functioning?

IV. **Thought Processes**

A. **Thought Form.** Thought form is the verbal record of how (not what) a patient is thinking. Normal thought form is logical and goal directed. A formal thought disorder may be characterized by circumstantiality or tangentiality, blocking, neologisms, clang associations, flight of ideas, and loose associations.

The physician should always record verbatim a brief extract of the patient's conversation to demonstrate the patient's thinking and how he or she associates and connects subjects. Is the train of thought logical and coherent? Can the patient's associations be followed easily? If the physician cannot do this, he or she should describe why.

B. **Thought Content.** Thought content refers to what the patient is thinking with less emphasis on the form or process. A great deal of the patient's thought content becomes apparent as the interview progresses. However, the physician may need to ask specific questions to clarify certain features. In addition to evaluating what the patient considers important, the interviewer must assess his reality testing by observing for delusions or other psychotic symptoms and asking specifically if the patient has ever had hallucinations. This is an appropriate place to determine if the patient has suicidal ideations or plans.

1. **Feelings of Unreality and Depersonalization**

    a. The phenomenon of dejà vu may be demonstrated by asking, "Did you ever have the feeling on entering a strange place that you had been there before?"

    b. Concerning other aspects of depersonalization one may ask, "Do persons and objects appear strange to you? Do you feel as if you are in a fog? Do you feel unnatural or as if your identity was lost? Is time or space distorted? Do you feel a change in yourself?"

2. **Feelings of Being Controlled**

    • Have you had any unusual, unpleasant, or perplexing experiences?
    • Have you had any peculiar thoughts, imaginations, or dreams?
    • Do you feel your thoughts or actions are controlled by others?
    • Do people read your mind?
    • Are your thoughts being taken away from you?
    • Is your mind or body influenced by machines, electricity, radio or television, mind reading, hypnotism, or telepathy?
    • Can you explain how such a thing could happen?

3. **Persecutory Trends.** If the patient's story seems suspicious, explore this by asking the following questions:

   - Are you considered friendly or popular?
   - Do you enjoy the company of others?
   - Do they treat you well?
   - Do people refer to you by changes in facial expression, side glances, or mumblings?
   - Do people gossip about you?
   - Do you find yourself seeing meanings in little things?
   - Are you a suspicious or jealous person?
   - Have you ever felt that strangers in the street were talking about you?
   - Have you ever felt that you were being wronged by someone, being annoyed by them purposely, or being robbed or poisoned?
   - How do you explain such occurrences?

4. **Obsessions and Compulsions (Fears).** These are common symptoms, and almost all patients are willing to talk about them freely. The physician should routinely ask the following questions:

   - Are you aware of thoughts of which you are unable to control or rid yourself?
   - Are you afraid of heights, crowds, small rooms, traffic, bridges, water or storms?
   - You know that children sometimes avoid stepping on the cracks in the sidewalk. Have you ever followed a ritual like that?
   - Have you ever felt tense if you did not follow one of these rituals?
   - What do they mean to you?

5. **Somatic Trends**

   - How is your health and strength?
   - Do you have any aches or pains?
   - How is your appetite, digestion, and excretory function?
   - Are you ever conscious of your heartbeat?
   - What is your level of sexual activity?
   - What does this mean to you?

6. **Expansive Trends**

   - Do you feel confident in yourself or superior to others?
   - Do you have unusual powers?

- Do you have a great physical strength, a brilliant mind, or tremendous wealth?
- Are you of high birth?
- Do you have a special mission in your life?
- Do you have great sexual attraction?

7. **Illusions**

- Have you ever found yourself misinterpreting shadows or noises?
- Did you ever feel you were being touched by something but nothing was there?
- Did you ever see a ghost?

8. **Hallucinations:** Patients should be asked these questions to determine if they are hallucinating with any of the five senses.

   a. **Auditory**

   - Do you hear buzzing in your ears or noises or voices that other people do not hear?
   - Where, when, and on what occasions?
   - Are they subdued or loud and clear?
   - Are they men's or women's voices?
   - Do you recognize them?
   - What do they say?
   - Are they pleasant or unpleasant?
   - How do you explain such happenings?
   - Are they telling you what to do?

   b. **Visual**

   - Did you ever see a vision?
   - Did you ever imagine you were seeing things as if in a dream?
   - Were your eyes open or shut?
   - Was it nighttime or daytime?
   - Where and when did they occur?
   - What feelings do you have when you see these things?
   - What does all of this mean?

   c. **Gustatory**

   - Does everything taste normal?
   - Have you noticed any peculiar tastes such as sour, bitter, or metallic?
   - Did your food ever taste as if it were being tampered with?

d. Olfactory

- Have you ever been bothered by strange odors?
- Have you smelled ether, gas, or smoke or as if something was burning?
- Have you been forced to bathe frequently?

e. Touch

- Do you ever feel any peculiar pressures, tingling, or numbness?
- Does your skin feel as if bugs are crawling on or under it?
- Do you ever feel as if your bones were broken or your brain had dried up?
- Do you ever feel any unusual sexual sensations?
- Have you ever had feelings of electricity or vibration?
- Did you ever notice any peculiar change in your body?
- Do you have strange sensations from muscles or joints?

V. Sensorium and Mental Capacity

A. Orientation. Determine how well the patient is oriented to time, place, person, and the present situation. In every record, all four points must be specifically mentioned.

B. Memory. The following subgroupings must be recorded.

1. **Recall of Remote Past Experiences.** Test the patient's recall of personal experiences (generally considered of importance) and evaluate discrepancies and contradictions in time relationships. Frequently, this information has already been obtained and recorded when the personal history was taken. In this case, the physician may merely refer to these facts. Patients should be tested with the time and place of their birth, various schools they attended, occupations or jobs they held, the date of their marriage, the date of birth and names of their children, and the date of their illness.

2. **Recall of Recent Past Experiences.** The physician should test for occurrences in the past 24 hours and whether a change in memory function has occurred since the onset of the present illness.

3. **Recall of Immediate Impressions.** The patient repeats three nonrelated words (e.g., table, red, 63 Broadway) and recalls them after 3 minutes. Present the patient with the three words, and tell the patient that you will

ask him or her to repeat them soon. Continue taking the patient's history, and after 3 timed minutes, ask the patient to recite the three words presented previously.

C. Attention and Concentration

1. **Digit Span.** The patient immediately repeats digits, starting with three digits and increasing until he or she fails to repeat them correctly. The physician records the number of digits correctly repeated. The physician repeats the digits one per second in an even tone of voice. It is important to avoid grouping or clustering digits, as in a telephone number. As a result of anxiety, patients often repeat two digits less than they would normally.

Digits Forward	Digits Backward
582	629
694	415
6439	3279
7286	4968
42731	15286
75836	61843
619473	539418
392487	724856
5917428	8129365
4179386	4739128
58192647	94376258
38295174	72819653
275862584	
713942568	

Highest Trial of Two Trials	
Digits Forward	Digits Backward
7 Good average	5 Average
6 Low average	4 Marginal
5 Marginal	

2. **Serial Subtraction.** Ask the patient to subtract 7 from 100 and continue subtracting by 7 until he or she can go no further. Record the results carefully and time the patient. Tension and anxiety may cause one or two mistakes; four to six errors are marginal; and seven errors or more constitute failure. The average time for the test is about 60 seconds.

D. General Intellectual Evaluation. The physician investigates a patient's knowledge to obtain a general understand-

ing of his intellectual functions and how he or she applies these functions to acquire information in school and in life. The following are suggested topics for a general intellectual evaluation.

1. **General Information**

   - What are the five largest cities in the United States?
   - What is the capital of this state, as well as the United States, England, France, and Germany?
   - When did the principal wars of the United States take place, and what issues were involved?
   - Who were the last four presidents and what were their political parties?
   - Who is the governor of the state and the mayor of the city in which you live?
   - Explain the seasons.
   - What is the gulf stream?

2. **Calculation.** Have the patient perform some simple calculations.

   - Compute 1½ years of interest at 4% on $200.
   - If five times X equals 20, how much is X?

3. **Symbolization.** Have the patient state the differences and similarities between abstract words such as idleness and laziness, ignorance and apathy, poverty and misery, character and reputation, and irresponsible and incapable.

4. **Proverb Interpretation:** Proverb interpretations test associations, abstraction, and the ability to symbolize and synthesize. These abilities are dependent on intelligence, education, culture, and the presence of organic defect and anxiety, but they are also dependent on the disturbed thought caused by schizophrenia.

VI. **Insight and Judgment.** Insight refers to the extent to which the patient realizes that he or she suffers from an illness or from personal difficulties and the extent to which he or she recognizes the need for treatment. Judgment is the patient's ability to make appropriate decisions about his or her life. According to individual needs, ask about the patient's plans for business and work, financial situations, and home and social situations.

MINI-MENTAL STATE EXAMINATION (MMSE)

The MMSE, developed by Folsein in 1975, is a standardized, quantified measure of sensorium and mental capacity (a portion of the mental status examination).[1] It is not an abbreviated version of the complete mental status examination. The outline below gives directions on how to perform and score the MMSE.

The physician says, "I am going to ask you a number of questions and ask you to do certain things to assess how well you are doing. Is that all right?"

Questions	Time Allowed for Response	Maximum Score
What year is this? (Accept exact answer only.)	10 sec	1
What season is this? (Accept either season if it is the last week of the old season or the first week of the new season.)	10 sec	1
What month is this? (Accept either month if it is the first day of the new month or the last day of the old month.)	10 sec	1
What is today's date? (Accept the previous or following date from the actual date.)	10 sec	1
What day of the week is this? (Accept exact answer only.)	10 sec	1
What country are we in? (Accept exact answer only.)	10 sec	1
What state are we in? (Accept exact answer only.)	10 sec	1
What city are we in? (Accept exact answer only.)	10 sec	1
What is the name of this building? (Accept exact answer only.)	10 sec	1
What floor of the building are we on? (Accept exact answer only.)	10 sec	1
I am going to name three objects or items. Remember them as I am going to ask you to repeat them later. (State all three items slowly for 1 sec each, then ask the patient to repeat them. The score, 1–3, is based on this first response. If needed, repeat the names of the objects a maximum of five times until the patient learns them or fails to do so.)	20 sec	3
Spell the word "world" backwards. (The score is the number of letters in the correct order.)	30 sec	5

[1] Folstein MF, Folstein SE, McHugh PR: Mini-mental state: a practical method for grading the cognitive state of patients. *Psych Res* 12:189–198, 1975.

(CONTINUED)

Questions	Time Allowed for Response	Maximum Score
Can you name the three objects I asked you to remember? (Give 1 point for each correct response regardless of the order given.)	10 sec	3
What is this object? (Show a wristwatch, and accept the correct answer only.)	10 sec	1
What is this object? (Show a pen or pencil, and accept the correct answer only.)	10 sec	1
Repeat this phrase after me, "no ifs, ands, or buts." (Accept the completely correct repetition only.)	10 sec	1
Read what this says, and do what it says. (Show the patient a sheet of paper on which the physician has written, "close your eyes." Ask the patient to do so up to three times.)	10 sec	1
Ask the patient if he or she is right- or left-handed, then hand him a piece of paper while saying, "Take this paper in your right (or left) hand, fold it in half, and put the paper on the floor." (Score 1 point for each activity done correctly.)	30 sec	3
Give the patient a pen and paper and say, "Write a sentence." Score if done.	30 sec	1
Give the patient a copy of the design below and say, "Please copy this design." (The patient must correctly draw two intersecting pentagrams with only two intersecting angles.)	60 sec	1

Maximum Total Score   30

Interpretation of the MMSE Score

Most people score a 30.

A score of 24–30 is within the normal range.

A score of 20–23 denotes some cognitive impairment, but the person can usually live independently.

A score of 20 or less denotes significant cognitive impairment with problems in living independently.

REPORTING THE MMSE

The physician should record the patient's score and then list the specific items missed.

DEFINITION OF TERMS

Affect is the *objective* expression of feeling or emotion. It encompasses all outward manifestations of the emotions that can be observed, including facial expression, gestures, posture, style of speaking (often culturally influenced), and motor activity. *Appropriate affect* is modulated by the situation or topic. An *inappropriate affect* is seen when the situation or topic and the observed expression of emotion are incongruent and often bizarre and disconcerting. The intensity or range of affect is described as normal, restricted, blunted, or flat as less and less expression occurs.

Alexithymia is the inability to describe emotions or feelings.

Anhedonia is the inability to enjoy anything; it is the opposite of hedonism. Anhedonia results in a loss of interest in and cessation of previously pleasurable activities.

Anxiety is apprehension, tension, or uneasiness stemming from the anticipation of danger from a largely unknown or unrecognized source. Anxiety is primarily intrapsychic in origin in contrast to fear, which is the emotional response to a consciously recognized and real external threat or danger. Anxiety and fear are accompanied by similar physiologic changes. Anxiety is considered pathologic when it interferes with conducting routine activities, the achievement of desired and realistic goals or satisfactions, or reasonable emotional comfort.

Apathetic describes the patient who shows a lack of interest, is indifferent, or lacks feeling.

Association is the relationship between ideas or emotions by contiguity, by continuity, or by similarities.

Autism (autistic thinking) is a form of thinking that reflects internal desires without regard for reality. Objective facts are distorted, obscured, or excluded in varying degree.

Blocking is difficulty in recollecting events or interruptions of a train of thought or speech resulting from (typically unconscious) emotional factors.

Circumstantial is a characteristic of a conversation that proceeds indirectly to its goal, with many tedious details and parenthetical and irrelevant additions.

Clang associations are associations that are governed by rhyming sounds rather than meaning, such as, "This what I thought, bought, knot, caught, rot, sought."

Compulsion is an insistent, repetitive, intrusive, and unwanted urge to perform an act that is contrary to the person's ordinary conscious wishes or standards. Anxiety results from the failure to perform the compulsive act.

Confabulation is the unconscious, defensive "filling in" of actual experiences that are recounted in a detailed, plausible, and often complex way as though they were factual.

Delusion is a false belief that does not match the individual's level of knowledge and his or her cultural group. The belief is maintained against logical argument and despite objective contradictory evidence. Common delusions include *delusions of grandeur* (exaggerated ideas of one's importance or identity), *delusions of persecution* (ideas that one has been singled out for persecution or punishment), and *delusions of reference* (incorrect assumption that certain casual or unrelated remarks or the behavior of others applies to oneself).

Dementia is decreased intellectual function with no decrease in consciousness.

Depersonalization is feelings of unreality or strangeness concerning either the environment or oneself.

Depression is a morbid sadness, dejection, or melancholy. It is differentiated from grief that is realistic and in proportion to what has been lost. A depression may vary from mild with little interference in functioning to psychosis.

Dissociation is a psychological separation or splitting off. It is an intrapsychic defensive process that operates automatically and unconsciously.

Echolalia is the repetition of words or phrases just spoken by someone else.

Echopraxia is the repetition of movements just made by someone else.

Euphoria is an exaggerated feeling of physical and emotional well-being inconsistent with apparent stimuli or events. It usually is psychological in origin but may be seen in organic brain disease and toxic states.

Flattened affect is characterized by a display of an abnormally small range of emotional expression.

Flight of ideas is speech that skips from one idea to another before the last one has been concluded. The ideas appear to be continuous but are fragmentary and determined by chance associations.

Hallucinations are false sensory perceptions in the absence of actual external stimuli. They may have an emotional or external chemical (drugs, alcohol) origin and may occur in any of the five senses.

Illusion is the misinterpretation of a real, external sensory experience.

Inappropriate affect is an emotional expression that is inconsistent with the situation or topic of discussion, such as giggling when talking about the death of a parent.

Insight is an accurate awareness of one's situation. A major goal of psychotherapy is for the individual to understand the origin, nature, and mechanisms of his or her attitudes and behavior. On a more superficial level, the patient recognizes that he or she is mentally ill.

Judgment is the complex process of assessing a situation and acting appropriately based on that assessment.

Loose associations occur when the normal connections or associations in the flow of thought are not present. They can range from circumstantial to tangential to incoherent.

Loss of goal is a failure to follow a chain of thought to its logical conclusion. It is usually elicited by asking a question; the patient starts to answer but then seems to wander off the subject.

Mood is the *subjective* emotional state of the patient; how the patient feels, described in his or her own terms. It can range from depressed (dysphoric) to normal (euthymic) to elevated (euphoric, ecstatic). It is best documented by directly quoting the patient's words.

Neologism is a new word or condensed combination of several words not readily understood by others. Neologism is common in schizophrenia.

Obsession is a persistent, unwanted idea or impulse that cannot be eliminated by logic or reasoning.

Orientation is an awareness of oneself in relation to time, place, person, and situation.

Perseveration (stereotypy) is the persistent, mechanical repetition of an activity. It is common in schizophrenia.

Phobia is an obsessive, persistent, unrealistic fear of an external object or situation such as heights, open spaces, dirt, or animals.

Pressure of speech is often rapid, difficult-to-interrupt speech that sounds like it is being pushed out rather than flowing normally.

Psychosis is a loss of touch with reality. It is caused by misinterpretation of sensory input or circumstances (delusions) or response to internal stimuli (hallucinations). It is a malfunction of cognitive, integrative higher functions or thought processes.

Sensorium roughly approximates consciousness. It includes the special sensory perceptive powers and their central correlation and integration in the brain. A clear sensorium indicates a reasonably accurate memory and correct orientation to time, place, and person.

Tangentiality is a disturbed thought process in which the patient never brings closure to the subject about which he or she is talking. The patient's thoughts begin sensibly but do not logically travel from point to point to closure.

Thought content is the focus of a person's thinking. Thought content ranges from normal to abnormal (delusions, obsessions).

Thought disorder is a disturbance in the process or form of thinking in contrast to the content of thought. It is the essence of psychosis.

Verbigeration is the meaningless repetition of words or phrases.

Word salad consists of an incoherent mixture of words and phrases. There is no association between words or phrases. Word salad indicates severe psychosis.

CHAPTER 3
Schizophrenia and Other Psychoses

Terry A. Travis, M.D., M.S.Ed.

SCHIZOPHRENIA

Definition

Schizophrenia is a chronic, severe mental illness characterized by a thought disorder. Other distinguishing features include delusions, hallucinations, behavior disturbances, and generalized deterioration in daily functioning.

Chief Complaint

- "I'm hearing voices telling me to do bad things."
- "Why are the aliens picking on me and trying to hurt me?"
- "Things keep happening to me that I do not understand."

Frequently, the patient's bizarre or nonsensical behavior prompts the family or school to have him or her evaluated.

Differential Diagnosis

Several causes must be ruled out. Stimulants, hallucinogens, cocaine, phencyclidine, and other street drugs can cause delusions, paranoia, and hallucinations. Alcohol withdrawal, acute neurologic conditions, head trauma, electrolyte imbalance, hyperthyroidism, and steroid use must be considered as well. Other psychiatric conditions should be considered, including mania in bipolar disorder, depression with psychosis, atypical and schizophreniform psychosis, and mental retardation. Any medical condition that affects brain function can cause psychotic symptoms resembling schizophrenia.

Screening

- Complete medical history and physical examination
- A complete blood count (CBC) and laboratory panel with electrolytes and thyroid function studies
- Neurologic studies as indicated
- Drug screens on both blood and urine

Diagnosis

To diagnose schizophrenia, two or more of the characteristic symptoms must be actively present for 1 month, and the signs and symptoms of disturbance of functioning must be present for at least 6 months. Patients with schizophrenia exhibit a decreased level of functioning in social relationships, work, and activities of daily living (ADLs) such as bathing and eating. Because of the implications about the severity of the illness and the response to medications, symptoms are often categorized as **positive** or **negative.** Positive symptoms mean that an active disordered process is occurring in the patient's mind. Negative symptoms mean that normal mental processes are dampened or turned off.

POSITIVE SYMPTOMS

Hallucinations are false sensory perceptions that occur with no external stimuli. Visual, auditory, tactile, taste, and olfactory hallucinations can occur. The most frequent hallucinations schizophrenic patients experience are auditory. The next most frequent are visual hallucinations. The physician must be alert for **command hallucinations,** voices that tell the patient to do something dangerous to him- or herself or others. Patients who report command hallucinations have a high incidence of acting on them, and active treatment and intervention are warranted.

Illusions are incorrect interpretations of a real stimulus. Most people have experienced this type of false sensory perception.

- **Clinical Questions.** The patient can be asked the following questions:
  - Are you seeing things that are not there?
  - Do you see or hear things that most people do not see or hear?
  - Do you have visions?
  - Do you hear voices?
  - What do they sound like?
  - What are they saying?
  - Can you identify to whom the voices belong?
  - Do you ever do things the voices tell you to do?
  - Can you tell me what you are seeing?
  - Are you experiencing sensations that other people do not have or would think unusual or abnormal?
  - What is your reaction to these voices or visions?
  - Are they frightening or pleasurable?
  - Do you ever smell, taste, or feel things that you cannot explain?
  - Can you tell me what is distracting you?
  - At what are you looking, and to what are you listening?

- **Clinical Observations.** Patients may be distracted by stimuli such as voices or visions that do not exist. They may look toward something you cannot see, appear to be listening to something, or their affect may change. The patient's facial expressions may show fear or happiness; he or she may smile, talk to, or respond to something the physician cannot understand or observe.

The physician should straightforwardly question patients concerning what is happening to them. Frequently, patients will respond by describing what they are perceiving and to what they are reacting.

Delusions are false beliefs often intertwined with the patient's perceptual disturbances (hallucinations) and disordered thoughts. Common delusions include:

- Persecution or paranoia: "The FBI is out to get me."
- Grandiosity: "I am God and am transforming the world."
- Somatic: "My organs are melting."
- Thought broadcasting: "Others know what I am thinking and can read my mind."
- Thought insertion: "Others are putting their thoughts into my mind."
- Ideas of reference: "The television show was telling me what to do."

- **Clinical Questions.** The patient should be asked the following questions:
  - Do you feel that you are being persecuted?
  - Do you have special talents or powers?
  - How is your thinking?
  - Are you having unusual thoughts?
  - Does the radio or television speak to or about you?
  - Is there anything happening to you that you do not understand?

- **Clinical Observations.** The physician should suspect the presence of delusional thought if the patient reacts strangely to routine questions during the history or physical examination. The patient may respond haughtily to the questions or demand to know why each question is being asked or why each part of the physical examination is taking place. The patient may refuse to respond to questions or may not allow the physical examination. This unusual behavior suggests that the patient is interpreting normal physician–patient interactions incorrectly. The physician should question this behavior to clarify its cause while remaining sensitive and sympathetic.

Behavioral disturbances range from wildly active, aggressive, and bizarre actions, termed agitated catatonia or catatonic rage, to complete inactivity, termed catatonic stupor. Occasionally, but not often, the behavior and thought disorder are connected, as in delusions and hallucinations.

Thought disorder, the quintessential symptom of schizophrenia, often accompanies hallucinations, delusions, and inappropriate behavior. The common terms that define the extent and severity of the thought disorder are circumstantiality, tangentiality, and looseness of association.

- **Circumstantiality.** Patients exhibiting circumstantiality mention unnecessary details and wander from the main topic, discussing events secondary to the topic. This style of thought is common and is considered minimally pathologic. The patient always returns to the primary topic and brings closure; the discussion just follows a long and deviating route where both logical connections and irrelevant details are seen. Patients who think and present information in this way say a great deal, but with little significant content. This often frustrates the clinician attempting to take the patient's history.

- **Tangentiality.** Tangentiality is clearly a pathologic disorder. Patients never bring closure to their ideas and do not perceive their thought as disordered. They often end up talking about something that has no connection to the topic originally under discussion.

- **Looseness of Association.** Derailment is the classic thought disorder of schizophrenia. The connections between sentences or between thoughts are absent. The clinician cannot follow, to varying degrees, the patient's thought process or understand what he or she is saying. This disorder can range from a subtle to a blatant thought disorder. When a subtle thought disorder is present, the physician will often feel that he or she knows what the patient is trying to express; however, the physician will find that he or she cannot write it down as a logical medical history. The most blatant thought disorder is termed a "word salad." Word salad exists when one is unable to understand connections from one word to the next, because the patient's speech is completely incoherent.

NEGATIVE SYMPTOMS

- **Blunting of emotions** manifests as an abnormal affect.
- **Mood** is the patient's description of how he or she feels. Affect is based on objective data from observations, while mood is determined by the patient's subjective report.
- **Affect** refers to the visible expressions of emotion that occur automatically, although they can be influenced by ethnic and cultural learning patterns. Physicians determine affect by observing physical clues such as posture, facial expressions,

gesticulations, eye contact, and general body movements. Schizophrenic patients exhibit a variety of abnormal affects:

- **Inappropriate**—smiling or giggling while talking about something sad or dangerous
- **Labile**—changing rapidly for no discernible reason
- **Range**—may be a noticeably restricted or blunted affect compared to that of a normal person.
- **"Flat affect"**—almost no emotional expression. These patients look like automatons, have no facial or body movements, and speak in monotones with no prosody (the normal rhythm and singsong quality of speaking).

- **Withdrawal.** This is a global withdrawal from interaction with others and from interest in the outside world. These patients focus on their internal thought processes and fantasies, while neglecting to interact with external reality.

- **Cognitive Deficits.** These overlap with withdrawal symptoms, as patients do not initiate goal-directed activity. This behavior interferes with the patient's ability to work and perform ADLs such as bathing, preparing meals, shopping, and planning ahead.

- **Poverty of Speech and Motor Activity.** The patient may sit without speaking or interacting for hours. When stimulated (such as being called to dinner), the patient will move normally (the opposite of catatonia). However, he or she does not initiate ongoing activities. While engaged in conversation, the patient's responses may be minimal, vague, or stereotypy. Conversation is often one-sided, since the patient says little or nothing.

CASE STUDY: YOUNG MAN WITH SCHIZOPHRENIA

A 23-year-old man had a chief complaint of, "I am just trying to get a job." When questioned about his attempts to work or get a job his answers gradually became more vague and tangential, especially when asked for more details. He began by giving reasonable responses, describing the kind of work he wanted, but he gave progressively vague reasons why nothing seemed to work or why a particular job was not appropriate for him. The examiner felt that the patient spoke convincingly but always had a vague excuse why he did not apply for or accept a job. These examples of loose associations and tangential thinking often frustrated the interviewer. In the past 2 years, the patient has never held a position for longer than 2 days. During that time, he also withdrew even further from his relationships, quit work for inexplicable reasons, and began talking about roommates and friends who made him uncomfortable or picked on him. His affect flattened, he exhibited increased inappropriate laughter and smiling, and his speech lost its normal prosody. The patient was never agitated. He was superficially cooperative but often passively broke promises by changing the recommended doses of medicine or decreasing his involvement in outpatient treatment programs. He was always neatly dressed and clean for appointments, but his case manager reported that he cleaned his room only when forced once a month. He did not bathe often and would wear the same clothes for several days. He would plan days ahead of time for appointments to be certain he had clean clothes and had bathed. He remained markedly superficial, only functioning when forced and participating passively in ongoing therapy. Occasionally, his paranoid ideation provoked feelings that people were planning things against him or that television shows had something to do with him. The patient was unable to provide an understandable explanation of what was happening. His thought processes became more loosely associated as he tried to clarify what was happening. He had been hospitalized twice, but with medication and regular social support has currently remained out of hospitals for more than 5 years. He has had to move three times as a result of "hassles with my roommates," and still talks of working but has done nothing about getting a job. He refuses to participate in any job training or preparation available, saying, "I do not need that, I am not that stupid." He has little insight, and demonstrates poor judgment.

Case Study: Homeless Man with Schizophrenia

A 36-year-old homeless man moved to the area "to be near a lawyer." No further history was obtained as a result of his markedly loose associations. When asked why he selected this town, the patient spoke of "the attorney general, stars overhead," and other nonsensical phrases. He was not interested in staying in a crisis bed, "I am on the corner and that is OK." He was dirty with marked body odor, had poor eye contact, and was mildly agitated, constantly moving about in his chair and standing up for no apparent reason. He was unable to describe any past treatment or any current medications except to say, "I have been to places like this before." The physician had to interrupt his talk of how everything—plots, television, air—centered around him, affected him, or tried to hurt him. He refused a physical examination but said he would take medication to "help me sleep." He often appeared to be attending to voices. He would stop talking for no apparent reason, scowl and focus his attention, occasionally mutter something indecipherable, and then resume talking. He accepted some samples of medication and was willing to meet with the chronic care team. The goal was to establish a relationship and provide follow-up care.

Case Study: Student with Schizophrenia

A 20-year-old college student was referred by her father who was concerned about "her obsessions and compulsions." The patient was neatly groomed and dressed. She was cooperative, maintained eye contact, and demonstrated a reasonable and appropriate range of affect. She described the increasing difficulties she faced in completing her college homework this year. She had had no problems during her first year of college. The problems consisted of her requiring more and more details before being able to start an assignment. Then, once started, she would spend days writing one page and feeling it was no good. She began speculating more often about such things as the need to bathe, how to bathe correctly, worrying about the soap, and how many towels to use. When she presented her history, it mimicked the typical onset of obsessions and compulsions. However, the more she talked, the more vague and abstract she became. Her philosophical ramblings, use of neologisms, and loose associations were not logical. After two 90-minute sessions, the physician ascertained that the obsessions and compulsions were a response to a psychotic thought process, not the increasing tension typical of obsessive-compulsive disorder. The patient had also withdrawn from friends and would often stay in her old room at home for 1–2 weeks to "work on my college assignments." She stated that her "worries about everything" had started 12–15 months previously. She was fairly insightful, both realizing she was not doing well and worrying about her future if she flunked out of college. The diagnosis was a first episode of psychosis, most likely schizophrenic versus psychosis not otherwise specified. Small doses of a neuroleptic medication decreased the symptoms by approximately 70%, but the patient was unable to return to college and cannot work as a result of disorganization and distrust of others.

Treatment

Research has shown that the most effective treatment includes both *psychosocial* and *biological* methods.

Psychosocial Therapies

All schizophrenic patients should be referred to a mental health center for care. There a treatment team includes a psychiatrist, trained counselors, psychologists, and social workers. Treatment focuses on establishing a therapeutic alliance between the patient and the treatment team. Therapy *supports* the patient by positively reinforcing success in daily activities while working with individuals to avoid harm or hospitalization. The patient's needs and ability to function determine the amount of support, which ranges from maintaining weekly to daily contact and helping the patient with housing, shopping, money management, and decisions. Family therapy is also important; support groups are available for the families of schizophrenics. These groups help the family understand what has happened to their loved one, how they can avoid unnecessary stressors, how to recognize early signs of relapse, and where they can go for help for themselves and their ill family member.

BIOLOGIC OR SOMATIC THERAPIES

Electroconvulsive therapy, or shock therapy, is used only when patients present with:

- Marked, dangerous agitation
- Active suicidal thoughts
- Excited or retarded catatonia

PHARMACOTHERAPY (NEUROLEPTICS OR ANTIPSYCHOTIC DRUGS)

Neuroleptics are divided into two groups, the typical neuroleptics, which are dopamine receptor antagonists, and the atypical neuroleptics, which are both serotonin and dopamine receptor antagonists (Table 3-1). The typical neuroleptics cause many side effects, including the development of tardive dyskinesia, and effectively reduce only the positive symptoms of schizophrenia. The atypical neuroleptics cause fewer side effects, do not cause tardive dyskinesia, and reduce both the positive and negative symptoms of schizophrenia. The atypical neuroleptic medications are currently the first choice for the treatment of psychoses.

Side Effects

- **Anticholinergic** side effects include dry mouth, constipation, difficulty urinating, blurred vision, and, occasionally, confusional states (at higher doses).
- α-**Adrenergic blockade** results in hypotension (problematic in the elderly), impotence, and failure to ejaculate.
- **Antihistaminic effects** cause sedation.
- **Dopaminergic blockade** causes galactorrhea, amenorrhea, impotence, weight gain, tardive dyskinesia, and the extrapyramidal syndromes.
- **Tardive dyskinesia** is a severe, often irreversible side effect that results in a disfiguring movement disorder. The involuntary movements, which are repetitive choreiform or athetoid,

Table 3-1
Antipsychotic Medications

Name	Adult Dosage Range (mg/d)	Side Effects
Typical		
Chlorpromazine (Thorazine)	50–2000	Low extrapyramidal
Thioridazine (Mellaril)	50–800	High anticholinergic,
Mesoridazine (Serentil)	100–400	sedation, and hypotension
Fluphenazine (Prolixin)	2–40	
Perphenazine (Trilafon)	8–64	
Trifluoperazine (Stelazine)	5–80	High extrapyramidal
Thiothixene (Navane)	5–60	Low anticholinergic,
Haloperidol (Haldol)	2–100	sedation, and hypotension
Loxapine (Loxitane)	20–250	
Molindone (Moban)	50–225	
Atypical		
Clozapine (Clozaril)	75–900	Weekly WBC monitoring Low extrapyramidal High sedation, anticholinergic, and hypotension
Risperidone (Risperdal)	1–6	
Olanzapine (Zyprexa)	10–20	Low on all side effects
Quetiapine (Seroquel)	300–400	
Injectible		
Fluphenazine (Prolixin) Decanoate	12.5–75 every 2 weeks	
Haloperidol (Haldol) Decanoate	50–300 every month	Side effects reduced

typically involve the lips and tongue. It can also affect movements of the extremities and trunk. High-risk factors include increased age of the patient and the total cumulative exposure to dopamine antagonists. No effective treatment exists other than prevention by minimizing the use of dopamine antagonists.

- **Extrapyramidal syndromes** are acute dystonias, akathisia, and pseudoparkinsonism. The discomfort these side effects cause is the main reason patients do not comply with their medication schedule.
  - **Acute dystonias** are spasms of the neck, tongue, oral, and facial muscles. Torticollis is a typical reaction.
  - **Akathisia** is a feeling of restlessness, usually in the lower legs, which results in purposeless movements. Patients may

move their legs around, stand up and pace, or walk in place. Patients describe this as an uncomfortable feeling in their leg muscles, as if they are tight or aching and movement will relieve the feeling. The feeling in their legs is similar to the aches caused by flu.

- **Pseudoparkinsonism** is indistinguishable from Parkinson's disease; patients exhibit pill-rolling hand tremors, flattened affect, slowed motor response, cogwheeling movements, and gait disturbance. Symptoms are greatly reduced with the anticholinergic agents benztropine (Cogentin, 1–6 mg/d), trihexyphenidyl (Artane, 2–10 mg/d), diphenhydramine (Benadryl, 50–300 mg/d), and biperiden (Akineton, 2–8 mg/d).

- **Neuroleptic malignant syndrome** is a relatively rare but potentially lethal side effect or illness. If left untreated, 20% of these patients die. Delirium, autonomic dysfunction, fever, and muscle rigidity are the cardinal symptoms. This syndrome should always be considered when a patient develops these symptoms. Treatment consists of administering dantrolene (Dantrium).

Incidence and Prevalence

The "lifetime prevalence rate" for developing schizophrenia in any population is 1%, based on the results of international cross-cultural studies. A strong genetic component has been demonstrated. The onset of schizophrenia occurs most often in men between 15 and 24 years of age and in women between 25 and 34 years of age. It is the most serious and disabling mental illness in the world; almost 40% of patients admitted to psychiatric hospitals are schizophrenic.

SCHIZOPHRENIFORM DISORDER

These patients have psychotic symptoms that are indistinguishable from schizophrenia. This provisional diagnosis is made when the patient is clearly psychotic for more than 1 month but less than 6 months. If the patient's psychosis fully resolves in less than 6 months, the diagnosis is confirmed. Good prognostic findings include an acute onset, confusion or perplexity at the height of the psychotic episode, normal function socially and at work prior to the onset, and the absence of abnormal affect.

The chief complaints of the patient, differential diagnosis, screening evaluation, and treatment are the same as for a schizophrenic patient.

The etiology of schizophreniform disorder is unknown. Once the patient has experienced a schizophreniform episode, there is an increased likelihood of similar episodes recurring. The longer an episode lasts, the greater the chance the patient will eventually develop schizophrenia.

SCHIZOAFFECTIVE DISORDER

The diagnosis of schizoaffective disorder has been controversial. Is it a separate mental disorder, an unusual bipolar disorder, a variant of schizophrenia, or does the patient have two major mental illnesses that overlap sometimes and appear independently at other times? The longitudinal course of the illness clarifies the diagnosis. The patient must experience concurrently clear-cut psychotic symptoms typical of schizophrenia and clear-cut symptoms of depression or mania. The patient must also have a history of at least 2 weeks of schizophrenic symptoms without significant symptoms of a mood disorder. Additionally, the patient must have experienced the symptoms of a mood disorder for a significant period of the illness. Conversely, patients presenting with predominantly schizophrenic symptoms who occasionally get depressed or elated are diagnosed with schizophrenia. Patients without psychotic symptoms except when depressed or manic should be diagnosed with a mood disorder with psychotic features.

Patients are screened for organic illnesses and other psychiatric illnesses the same way as for schizophrenia and depression. The etiology is unknown. Treatment is based on symptomatology. Psychotic symptoms are treated with neuroleptics, and depressive or manic patients are treated with antidepressants or mood stabilizers.

DELUSIONAL DISORDERS

Patients with a delusional disorder exhibit no signs or symptoms of schizophrenia other than delusions. This is clearly not a subtype of schizophrenia. The delusions typically are well organized, internally consistent, and not bizarre. These patients function normally and effectively, except when their delusional concerns become involved. They have little insight into their illness and feel strongly about their beliefs, even if they appear blatantly false to others. These patients seem to present logical stories, if one can accept the critical belief upon which the story is based. Since the patient is passionate about his or her beliefs, the clinician must maintain a professional distance so as not to be drawn in.

The differential diagnosis and screening procedure are the same as for any other psychosis. Many medical disorders and substance abuse problems can present with significant delusions.

Delusional disorders are further classified as specific delusional disorders.

Specific Delusional Disorders

EROTOMANIA

Patients with erotomanic delusions believe that another individual, often of higher social status, is deeply in love with them. The patient may communicate inappropriately with the individual (the target of the delusional system), and the patient also may misinterpret the person's normal public behavior.

CASE STUDY: YOUNG WOMAN WITH AN EROTOMANIC DELUSIONAL DISORDER

A 19-year-old female nursing student was referred by her supervisor because she was missing classes and "paying too much attention to one of the psychiatrists in the clinic." The patient related that the psychiatrist was deeply in love with her, even though they had never talked alone. She had only heard him lecture or give a presentation two or three times. The patient knew he loved her because of where he parked his car in the hospital parking lot. She could state the exact time and location of where he parked and felt that it was a message of his love for her. The patient was aware that they had never talked, probably would never have a relationship, and that he was happily married. She was doing well in the nursing program except for tardiness to lecture and teaching activities because she was watching for the physician's arrival in the parking lot. She would also leave unsigned messages on his desk. Her mental status was normal except for this belief. The patient refused treatment, stating she did not want to embarrass him. She planned to get her nursing degree and then move away from him to find someone who could return her love.

GRANDIOSE DELUSIONAL DISORDER

Patients with grandiose delusional disorder believe they have special powers or abilities and may spend much of their time working on schemes, inventions, or documents that will benefit everyone.

CASE STUDY: MAN WITH GRANDIOSE DELUSIONAL DISORDER

The patient was a 48-year-old man who spent his working hours writing an abstruse, complicated philosophical theory that united mankind's religious and scientific beliefs. He had paid to have these works published, was developing a home page on the Internet, and had business cards printed. He functioned poorly at work because he was constantly thinking about his writings, but the patient was able to maintain himself financially.

Jealous Delusional Disorder

Jealous delusional disorder is the patient's belief that his spouse or lover is being unfaithful. This belief is supported by clues or evidence that the patient finds in random events, words used in conversation, or unaccounted time.

Case Study: Man with Jealous Delusional Disorder

A husband accused his wife of infidelity over the past 2 years, during which time he claimed she often met or contacted her lover. According to the patient, this was substantiated by phone calls he received once or twice where the caller claimed he had dialed the wrong number or the caller said he was sorry and hung up. This had occurred twice in the preceding year. The patient's wife was afraid to talk to him as he would interpret words or phrases as implying a relationship. Her silence only confirmed his suspicions. He constantly checked the mileage on her car and insisted on knowing everything she was doing and where she was going each day. He would drive the route he felt she should use, and if her mileage was off by one- or two-tenths of a mile he would accuse her of lying and claim that she had had a tryst with her lover. His wife denied ever having an affair. She was terrified of him, as he had threatened to kill her and her lover if he ever found them together. He would not give her a divorce and controlled all aspects of their lives. His wife knew of no precipitating event and reported that the first 5 years of their marriage had been fine. The husband refused to enter into therapy or receive treatment.

Persecutory Delusional Disorder

Patients suffer from persecutory delusional disorder when they feel that a specific organized plot is aimed at them or someone close to them. They may feel they are being followed or that their phone is tapped. These irrational beliefs often appear plausible if one can accept the premise. No thought disorder other than the specific persecutory delusional belief is present.

Somatic Delusional Disorder

Patients with somatic delusional disorder have the false belief that they have a specific physical defect or medical condition that has never been properly diagnosed. These conditions or defects may consist of infections from insects or parasites, the emission of odors from the body, organ dysfunction (i.e., liver, intestine, lung), or some physical defect. This is differentiated from somatization disorders by the delusional extent of the belief, but the diagnoses clearly overlap.

CASE STUDY: WOMAN WITH SOMATIC DELUSIONAL DISORDER

A 47-year-old woman had been hospitalized repeatedly with the belief that she had a magnesium deficiency that was making her feel ill all of the time. She had printouts from several medical school libraries of searches she had done on medical databases; hundreds of reprints of articles from journals from the fields of medicine, toxicology, environmental research, and engineering; and copies of newspapers and magazines. She would highlight a sentence in the middle of an article and misinterpret it so that it supported her beliefs. The woman did not respond to medication or psychotherapy and spent most of her time focused on and working to prove her belief. She functioned well enough to control her finances and her appearance and revealed no thought disorder or psychosis other than this belief.

MIXED DELUSIONAL DISORDER AND UNSPECIFIED DELUSIONAL DISORDER

When the criteria for delusional disorder are met but the delusions do not fit the specific subtypes described above, the patient is diagnosed with mixed delusional disorder or unspecified delusional disorder.

Treatment

Since medications generally give unsatisfactory results, the patient should be referred to a psychiatrist. Occasionally, neuroleptics or antidepressants are helpful, but often there is only a minimal response. The first treatment goal is to establish an ongoing relationship of trust with the patient. This is often a difficult and uncertain task.

BRIEF PSYCHOTIC DISORDER

Brief psychotic disorder is an acute psychotic episode in an otherwise normal individual, often precipitated by a stressful life event such as sudden severe physical disability, divorce, financial setbacks, or an accident. At least one of the following must be present to meet the diagnosis: delusions, hallucinations, disorganized or catatonic behavior, and disorganized speech. The onset is sudden, and the illness lasts at least 1 day but less than 1 month. The symptoms often disappear rapidly and dramatically. The differential diagnosis and screening procedures are the same as for any other psychosis.

Treatment

Treatment involves thoroughly assessing the risk of suicidal or homicidal ideation and carefully administering neuroleptics to control agitation and psychotic symptoms. Neuroleptic medications are only used for a short time and should be stopped soon after symptoms subside and the patient returns to baseline functioning. Psychotherapy should focus on recounting the events that precipitated the psychosis, while clarifying their meaning and significance for the patient. The goals are to help the patient learn and grow from the experience, minimize similar stressors in the future, and develop better coping mechanisms.

SHARED PSYCHOTIC DISORDER

Shared psychotic disorder is an unusual condition in which one person fully accepts the delusional beliefs of another person, usually either a family member or someone with whom he or she has had an extended intimate relationship. The dominant person usually suffers from schizophrenia or a delusional disorder, and the passive person has accepted and joined in the delusional system. Prior to becoming involved in the psychotic partner's psychosis, the passive person was not psychotic. In fact, the passive person often stops believing in the delusional system once he or she is separated from the dominant, sicker person. The submissive dependent partner has accepted the psychosis as a compromise to maintain the relationship with the dominant partner. The dominant individual needs treatment for the mental illness from which he or she is suffering. Following separation from the dominant person, the only treatment required for the dependent partner is rational discussion to orient him or her to reality.

CHAPTER 4
Mood Disorders

Terry A. Travis, M.D., M.S.Ed.

INTRODUCTION

Definition

Abnormal feelings that range from suicidally unhappy to grandiose. Both ends of the spectrum include psychotic thinking. Intermediate stages of abnormal feelings range from depression to sadness to unhappiness to feeling alright to being up to feeling high or hypomanic and, ultimately, to mania. There are several diagnoses within the mood disorders that encompass this entire range of feelings. Each requires distinct histories of episodes of major depression, mania, or hypomania or mixed episodes with both manic and depressive symptoms (Table 4-1). A **major depressive disorder** means that only depression is present. If a manic episode occurs, it is a **bipolar I disorder.** When there is a history of depression and a hypomanic episode occurs, it is termed a **bipolar II disorder. Dysthymia** is distinguished by a longstanding history of depressive symptoms that fail to meet the criteria for a depressive episode. When the cycles of depressive symptoms are not severe enough to meet the criteria for a depressive episode and alternate with hypomanic episodes, **cyclothymia** is diagnosed. If there are short-term symptoms of depression clearly related to a life event, this is termed an **adjustment disorder with depressed mood.** A "double depression" can occur when a patient who suffers from dysthymia also experiences a major depressive episode.

Chief Complaint

- "I just do not feel right."
- "Nothing seems important or interesting anymore."
- "Everything bothers me. I get really angry and upset easily."
- "I cannot do my work."
- "I feel tired, worn-out all the time."
- "I feel sad and depressed and cry for no reason."
- "I must be losing my mind, I cannot remember or finish anything."
- "All I think about is how terrible everything is, including myself."
- "I do not feel that there is any reason to go on anymore."

TABLE 4-1
DIAGNOSES AND SYMPTOMS OF MOOD DISORDERS

Symptom	Major Depressive Disorder	Bipolar I Disorder	Bipolar II Disorder	Dysthymia	Cyclothymia	Adjustment Disorder with Depressed Mood
Depression	X					
Mania		X	X			
Hypomania		X	X			
Mild depression				X	X	
Specific stressor					X	X

Differential Diagnosis

The following must be ruled out prior to making a psychiatric diagnosis:

- Neurologic disorders such as dementias, stroke, epilepsy, Huntington's disease, sleep apnea, Parkinson's disease, multiple sclerosis, and neoplasms
- Other medical conditions such as cancers of the pancreas and gastrointestinal system, cardiopulmonary disease, and renal disease
- Infectious diseases such as acquired immunodeficiency syndrome (AIDS), pneumonia, mononucleosis, tuberculosis, arthritis, and systemic lupus erythematosus (SLE)
- Diseases of the endocrine system, including Cushing's disease, hypo- and hyperthyroidism, and hypo- and hyperparathyroidism
- Drugs such as opiates, antibacterials, beta-blockers, clonidine, reserpine (many cardiac drugs), antineoplastics, hypnotics, steroids, cimetidine, stimulants, alcohol, and sedatives

The physician must take a complete medical history and perform a thorough physical examination. The following tests should be performed: a complete blood count (CBC) with hemoglobin and hematocrit levels, laboratory panels with thyroid function studies and electrolytes, urinalysis, electrocardiogram (ECG), and chest radiographs. Neurologic studies should be done if required.

Diagnostic Descriptors

A list of descriptors that can be added to the diagnosis of any episodes of depression or mania appears below.

- **Mild.** Minimal symptoms present to make the diagnosis; often difficult to separate from a dysthymic or hypomanic episode.
- **Moderate.** Clear-cut symptoms with some functional impairment; often the patient is functioning on a day-to-day basis.
- **Severe without Psychotic Features.** Marked symptoms, more than enough to meet criteria; significant impairment of function.
- **Severe with Psychotic Features.** Delusions, hallucinations, or both are present that can be mood congruent or mood incongruent. Function is severely impaired.
- **In Partial Remission.** Some symptoms are still present, and functioning is greatly improved.

- **In Total Remission.** No significant symptoms present for at least 2 months.
- **Catatonic Features.** At least two of the following are exhibited:
    Motoric immobility with catalepsy, waxy flexibility, or stupor
    Purposeless excessive activity
    Mutism or negativism
    Bizarre posturing, movements, mannerisms, or grimacing
    Echolalia or echopraxia
- **Melancholic Features.** Exhibited with:
    Anhedonia
    Expression of distinctly depressed mood
    Depression in the morning with improvement as the day progresses
    Early morning awakening
    Marked psychomotor slowing or agitation
    Significant loss of appetite and weight loss
    Guilt that is excessive and inappropriate
- **Atypical Features.** Exhibited with:
    Mood still reactive to events
    Increased appetite and weight
    Sensitivity to interpersonal rejection, socially or occupationally
    Feeling as if extremities are extremely heavy, leaden
- **Seasonal Pattern.** During the past 2 years there have been two episodes with the onset temporally related to a specific season; full remission occurs with the change of season.
- **Rapid-cycling.** When four episodes have occurred within 12 months.
- **Postpartum Onset.** When the onset is within 4 weeks of delivery.

SPECIFIC MOOD DISORDERS

Major Depressive Disorder

DIAGNOSIS

A diagnosis of major depressive disorder is made when one or more major depressive episodes have occurred. An episode must consist of at least **five** of the following symptoms (criteria) over a 2-week period.

1. **Criterion.** A depressed mood is exhibited most of the time.
    - **Clinical Questions.** How depressed are you? Do you feel sad most of the time? Do you feel empty or that there is no meaning to anything? When did you last feel all right? Do other people comment that you look sad or down?

- **Clinical Observations.** The patient shows no change in facial expression or posture. He or she appears sad throughout the interview.

2. **Criterion.** Anhedonia is a lack of pleasure in everything or in most activities.
    - **Clinical Questions.** Do you enjoy doing anything? Are there things in the past you enjoyed doing, such as activities, hobbies, movies, reading, playing with the kids, that you find no pleasure in now? What can you get into now and enjoy? How is your interest in and enjoyment of sex? Tell me about something you particularly enjoy and how much you enjoy it now.
    - **Clinical Observations.** There is no observed change or modulation in affect.

3. **Criterion.** A change in appetite is seen. Appetite either decreases or increases, with or without a concomitant change in weight. Anhedonia can also affect appetite.
    - **Clinical Questions.** How is your appetite? Do you eat just because you have to or do you enjoy the food? Do you look forward to a meal or eating a food you really like? Has there been any weight change? How much? Do your clothes fit the same?

4. **Criterion.** There is a change in sleep pattern.
    - **Clinical Questions.** Tell me how you sleep? What is a typical night like for you? Do you have trouble going to sleep, or do you toss and turn all night? Do you wake up before you want to, such as at the end of the night or early in the morning, and cannot go back to sleep? Do you feel rested or tired and worn-out in the morning? Do you spend hours in bed beyond what you normally would? Does this help you feel rested or have more energy?
    - **Clinical Observations.** The patient appears tired. He or she yawns and looks drowsy.

5. **Criterion.** A change is noted in the patient's activity level. He or she may exhibit psychomotor agitation or retardation.
    - **Clinical Questions.** Do you feel keyed up or easily irritated? Do you feel tense all the time and cannot sit still? Do things bother you that normally would not, such as your kids, people at work, or background noises that you would usually ignore? Do you wonder why you respond with such anger or irritability and feel bad about your unusual behavior? (Agitation is often the symptom that causes the family or spouse to insist that the patient do something to get better, because the anger and irritability affect the entire family.) Do you feel slowed

down? Do you find that you want to do something but it takes a long time to finish it or that you have thought of doing something but are still just sitting and have not done anything yet? Do you feel sluggish, as if you have to push yourself to do anything? Does it feel as if everything you do is like pushing through a bowl of jelly? For example, you get it done but it takes lots of energy and you have to push yourself constantly.

- **Clinical Observations.** The patient has a delayed response to questions, which may last anywhere from a few seconds to 1 minute or more in severe cases. All motions are slower, including shifting while in the sitting position, walking into the room, and writing. When agitated, these patients can appear anxious. They pace, are unable to sit still or remain sitting, wring their hands, shift position frequently, and are curt and irritable when answering questions or giving their history.

6. Criterion. Fatigue and a lack of energy are seen. This symptom is similar to psychomotor retardation and feeling tired or unrested.

- **Clinical Questions.** How is your energy level? Are you always feeling tired and worn-out? Do you have to push yourself to do things? Do you feel like you are sick with the flu, aching, and just wanting to stay in bed? (This symptom is often the one that brings patients to their primary care physician to find out what is physically wrong with them. This symptom can also result in the patient staying in bed for several days.)
- **Clinical Observations.** The patient appears tired and may have psychomotor retardation.

7. Criterion. Feelings of worthlessness, hopelessness, helplessness, or inappropriate guilt are seen.

- **Clinical Questions.** How do you feel about yourself? Do you feel helpless or hopeless? (These feelings and thoughts can be of delusional severity.) Do you feel you have been an evil person? Do you feel condemned? Do you feel others would be better off without you? (Such feelings obviously lead to suicidal ideation [see below].)

8. Criterion. There is a decreased ability to concentrate or make decisions.

- **Clinical Questions.** Are you able to concentrate? Can you complete tasks or do you lose track of what you are doing? Can you read books or the newspaper and follow what you are reading? Can you get into and follow a television show? (Occasionally, concentration decreases to the point where the patient cannot read a newspaper article or attend to what is occurring in a movie or television show.) Do you still watch television shows you enjoy? If not, why not? (Clearly, an-hedonia and decreased concentration overlap in symptomatol-ogy.) Can you make decisions such as what to wear, what to eat, and what to do, or do you find yourself unable to make a decision and move on in the way you normally would? Does it matter to you what you do, eat, or wear?

- **Clinical Observations.** The patient may lose track of what he or she is answering and ask for the question to be repeated or may ask "what were we talking about?"

9. Criterion. The patient has thoughts of death or suicide. **If depression is being considered in the differential diagnosis, the physician must ask about suicide.** Most patients are comfort-able answering such questions and actually are comforted by the physician's concern. If the patient answers positively to questions about suicide, the physician should determine the following three things. Have they attempted suicide before and, if so, how many times? Second, do they have a specific plan to commit suicide? Finally, how lethal have their past attempts been, or how lethal are their current plans?

- **Clinical Questions.** Have you ever thought of suicide? How badly do you or have you felt? Have you wondered if it was worth going on? Have you wished you were dead? Have you wished that something would happen to end what you are going through or to take you away from everything? Do you or have you ever thought of suicide or of hurting or killing yourself? Have you ever done anything to hurt or try to kill yourself? What have you thought of doing? Have you done anything to prepare to kill or hurt yourself, such as collecting pills, turning the car toward a bridge support, turning a knife or gun on yourself, or going to a high place where you could jump into a river or traffic? Have you attempted suicide be-fore? If so, what did you do? How close are you now to killing yourself? Do you have any reason or situation that keeps you from killing yourself?

10. Criterion. The patient cries. Although this is not listed in the *Diagnostic and Statistical Manual of Mental Disorders*, 4th ed. *(DSM-IV)*, this symptom is often present and needs to be evaluated.

- **Clinical Questions.** Do you have crying spells? Do you feel like crying? When you feel like crying or do cry is there a reason? Are you thinking of or remembering something sad that makes you cry? Do you burst out in tears spontaneously for no obvious reason? Do you wonder why you do not under-stand what is happening when you cry?
- **Clinical Observations.** Patients may tear up or burst into

tears during the interview. The crying episode may or may not be related to the ongoing interview.

Many of the symptoms that comprise a depressive episode overlap, and there is a wide range of severity within and among the symptoms. All of this should be taken into account when obtaining the patient's history and while observing the patient as part of establishing a diagnosis. With clinical experience, the physician develops a feeling for the range of symptoms that patients experience. This enables the physician to evaluate the patient in-depth to reach a diagnosis.

CASE STUDY: MAN WITH A MAJOR DEPRESSIVE DISORDER

A 28-year-old single man presents with the chief complaint "I just don't feel well. I'm not interested in anything, have burst out in tears in the car, and am having problems doing my work." The interview reveals that he is sleeping poorly, tossing and turning and then awakening an hour early without being able to go back to sleep. He began exhibiting some symptoms 3-4 months ago. He cannot concentrate at his new job of 6 months or even follow an hour of television. He is not enjoying his usual interests. For example, he has stopped bowling regularly. His girlfriend feels that he is not interested in her because he wants to make love only once a month rather than 2-3 times a week. He has not lost weight but states, "I eat because I know I should. I am really not interested in food and do not look forward to meals." He feels like he has no energy and has wondered if life is really worthwhile but has no specific suicidal ideations or plans. Other than the new job, to which he had looked forward, he has no other stressors. His brother and an uncle both have been treated for depression, but no one in his family has attempted suicide.

TREATMENT

Antidepressants

Of those patients who experience a major depressive disorder, 65%-75% have a good response to antidepressants. All antidepressants are essentially equivalent in their effectiveness. Drug selection is often based on the side effects.

All antidepressants take 2-4 weeks to reach maximum therapeutic effect. However, if some of the depressive symptoms are not relieved after the first week, a higher dose is usually indicated. Patients should be told to continue taking the medication for the first 2 weeks even if relief is minimal. This allows the dosage to be adjusted. Side effects frequently occur within the first 1–3 days and are the only reason an antidepressant is stopped before sufficient time and dosage is reached.

Tricyclics such as imipramine, amitriptyline, nortriptyline, and doxepin were the first group of antidepressant medications. They cause many side effects that are, at minimum, uncomfortable and possibly dangerous. These include dry mouth, blurred vision, constipation, dizziness, and sedation. They should *not* be used with geriatric patients, since the risk of falls is high as a result of postural hypotension, and cardiac arrhythmias can be fatal. The tricyclics can be lethal because of their effects on the cardiac conduction system. Death from an overdose is usually the result of cardiac arrhythmia.

Many new antidepressants with low lethality and minimal side effects are now available. These antidepressants, the first choice in the treatment of depression, include the selective serotonin-reuptake inhibitors (SSRIs) [fluoxetine, sertraline, paroxetine]. Other new antidepressants include venlafaxine, nefazodone, and mirtazapine. Other, unique medications that have been available for some time are amoxapine, bupropion, and maprotiline.

MAOIs (monoamine oxidase inhibitors) such as phenelzine and tranylcypromine should only be used in special circumstances or when other antidepressants fail. Patients taking these medications must follow a special low-tyramine diet, as a hypertensive crisis can result when certain foods are eaten or when other medications are taken concurrently. MAOIs should be taken under the guidance of a psychiatrist.

Electroconvulsive Therapy (ECT)

This is the safest and most effective treatment for major depression. However, it is used only when antidepressant medications fail, when the patient is actively suicidal and it is too risky to wait for the antidepressant to take effect, or when there are medical conditions that contraindicate using antidepressants. There is no absolute contraindication other than increased intracranial pressure. ECT is effective in almost 95% of patients, and no side effects are seen except short-term confusion and the loss of immediate memory around the time of the treatments.

Psychotherapy and Counseling

Counseling should always be integrated with somatic therapies. This helps patients to cope with the effects of their illness, provides support for their families, and offers treatment for conflicts or issues that may have contributed to the onset of the depression. Medication and ECT do not erase the problems these patients have, and it is poor practice not to provide them with appropriate therapy.

EPIDEMIOLOGY

Fifteen percent of patients who are depressed for longer than 1 month commit suicide. Since this is the most lethal of the psychiatric illnesses, patients must always be probed for any suicidal ideations, plans, or attempts. Women have twice the lifetime risk for major depression as men (20%–26% vs. 8%–12%). Up to 20% of patients who have had an acute episode of major depression develop a chronic depressive syndrome.

Dysthymia

DIAGNOSIS

The patient must exhibit, for at least 2 years, a consistently depressed mood most of the time that is clearly *less* severe than that of a major depressive disorder. The chronic depressive illness typically starts in childhood or adolescence. These patients often complain of being depressed their entire lives. They may experience superimposed episodes of major depression and then suffer from what is termed a "double depression."

CASE STUDY: WOMAN WITH DYSTHYMIA

A 42-year-old married woman presents with the chief complaint, "I have always been depressed, as long as I can remember, it is just worse now." She reports that she has never really felt like she has enjoyed much of anything, but she is able to gain pleasure from her favorite television shows, music, her children, and reading. Recently she has had difficulty reading because she has lost the ability to concentrate. She sleeps well except when worried about her children or finances, which are not current issues. She has always "cried easily at any sad or sentimental film or seeing something on television that anyone would feel sad about." Her energy level is basically fine, and she has maintained her usual activities at home with her family, and at work. However, she reports that she has always had to push herself to get it all done. She has never felt suicidal. The patient was referred by her primary care physician, who had completed a full physical examination and basic laboratory studies that ruled out endocrine, hematologic, and other disorders.

TREATMENT

It is well known that a significant percentage (30%–60%) of patients with dysthymia respond to antidepressants; thus, a therapeutic trial is always indicated. There is no way to predict who will respond to medication. When a response occurs, it is often striking. Patients make comments such as, "So this is how most people feel," "I never knew that life could be so wonderful and I could feel what I feel," or "I've never felt this good in my life." Cognitive therapy and short-term focused psychotherapy are effective in helping dysthymic patients to recognize and change their distorted world views and to interpret interactions in less consistently pessimistic or negative ways. A trial of medication should, therefore, be administered, but psychotherapy is the principal treatment.

EPIDEMIOLOGY

Dysthymia occurs in approximately 6% of people during their lifetime. The prevalence is somewhat higher in women. Evidence has shown that a subgroup of dysthymic patients may be experiencing a less severe form of a major depressive disorder and are likely the same patients who respond to antidepressant medication.

Adjustment Disorder with Depressed Features

DIAGNOSIS

Depressive symptoms occur in response to an identifiable stressor in the patient's life. A relationship must be established to a psychosocial stressor. In adjustment disorder with depressed mood, the symptoms must start within 3 months of the beginning of the stressor, cannot continue longer than 6 months, and must continue after the stressor is gone. The depressive symptoms do not meet the criteria for either a major depressive episode or a dysthymic disorder.

CASE STUDY: MAN WITH ADJUSTMENT DISORDER WITH DEPRESSED FEATURES

A 50-year-old man presents with the chief complaint, "Since I was laid off work I am just not myself." A thorough history reveals no previous mood problem, and his symptoms began within the first 2 weeks after being laid off and have persisted for the past 3 months. He was laid off when his firm downsized. He has a small pension but cannot find work. He is tearful when he mentions his frustrations and concerns about his financial future and the effect this will have on friends and family. However, the patient enjoys doing things he has always done with friends, makes love with his wife as frequently and pleasurably as before, and enjoys family gatherings. He experiences no suicidal ideation but is angry about what has happened to him. He is actively looking for work and is able to make decisions. He has good concentration and sleeps well, except when he applies for a job and is rejected.

TREATMENT

Short-term crisis-oriented individual psychotherapy is the most commonly recommended treatment. Occasionally brief family therapy also helps. Self-help groups are often very helpful in providing peer support and sharing coping strategies. Medications should be used only for a short period of time to treat marked sleep disturbances or episodes of anxiety. They should be given on an as needed (prn) basis, and the physician should clearly explain that they will not solve the problem and are for short-term use only. Antidepressants should not be given as a response can take 3–4 weeks, and the symptoms best treated by the antidepressants are by definition not present.

BIPOLAR DISORDERS

The diagnosis of bipolar disorder I is made once an episode of mania has occurred. Bipolar disorder II is made when depressive episodes and hypomanic episodes occur.

Mania with or without Psychosis

DIAGNOSIS

Patients must exhibit at least three of the following symptoms of a persistently elevated or irritable mood for a minimum of 1 week.

1. Criteria. The patient has feelings of elation, increased self-esteem and grandiosity, or irritability.
- **Clinical Questions.** How good do you feel? Do you feel you can do anything or accomplish anything you want? Do you feel you are all powerful?
- **Clinical Observations.** The patient only talks about him- or herself and is very obviously grandiose.

2. Criterion. The patient has much less need for sleep. He or she often needs no sleep or only 2–4 hours a night for several nights.
- **Clinical Questions.** Has there been any time when you did not need much sleep or went for several days without sleep or only minimal sleep? Did you have more energy than usual even without sleeping? Did you wake up after a short time full of energy?

3. Criterion. The patient is very talkative with pressure of speech.
- **Clinical Questions.** Have you experienced times when you could not stop talking and the words just kept coming on their own?
- **Clinical Observations.** Pressure of speech is not necessarily related to the speed of speech, but it is often rapid. It refers to the feeling that the patient's words just keep coming as if something is behind them, pushing them out. This often makes it very hard to interrupt the manic individual. The patient may not be able to stop talking, even for brief periods

of time. The physician often gets the feeling that the patient is spitting the words out or having trouble keeping up with what he or she is saying.

4. Criterion. The patient feels that his or her thoughts are racing. Flight of ideas may be present in the patient's conversation.

- **Clinical Questions.** Has there been any time when your thoughts were racing out of control or going so fast that you could not keep up with them?
- **Clinical Observations.** While speaking, the patient shifts from one topic to another rapidly, although there is often at least a minimal connection between ideas. Conversely, with loose associations the patient shifts from topic to topic with no connection or sense whatsoever. The physician often feels as if he or she can barely keep up with the patient's conversation and that the patient "is all over the place." For example, the patient may say "Hi! I am ready to leave. Dame Margot Fonteyn is dancing in New York City tonight, and I have to catch a plane. Flying is really wonderful, and dancing is better. Have you ever seen her? I sometimes get tense on planes. I take lithium, but I am okay now and I hope I can see her. I have not seen you as my doctor before but I will later. Bye!" All this was said in 5 seconds by a patient who appeared at the physician's door and left. The physician had never seen him before. This is a good example of flight of ideas.

5. Criterion. The patient exhibits distractibility.

- **Clinical Questions.** Do you have trouble staying on one topic? Are you distracted by things going on around you? Do you find that you can not finish one thought before another enters your mind? Do you find yourself trying to do several things at the same time? Is your concentration really bad?
- **Clinical Observations.** The patient changes the focus of the conversation based on stimuli that normally would not be a distraction. For example, sounds heard or things seen in the room often lead to flight of ideas. The patient may say, "I'm glad to see you today. That is a really nice tie you have on. This room is too hot, but the walls are nicely painted and could use some decorations. The truck outside sure is loud but probably is picking up garbage. It sounds like my mother is just outside the door. Is your chair comfortable? My back hurts in bad chairs."

6. Criterion. Just the opposite can occur with an increased focus on one goal-directed activity such as work, social activities, sex, or other pleasurable activities.

- **Clinical Questions.** Have you found yourself being involved excessively in work (putting in 16–20-hour days) or other activities you really enjoy such as listening to music, watching sports on television, or making love with your partner? Have other people complained that you are overdoing the things you are involved in?
- **Clinical Observations.** The patient talks on and on about only one activity. For example, one patient talked only about spreading the American flag all around the country, in every square mile. Others involved with the patient report excessive interest and involvement in one activity. The patient's partner may complain that the patient wants to make love repeatedly to the extent that sleep deprivation occurs.

7. Criterion. The patient does things that are pleasurable that he or she later regrets or that may result in a great deal of embarrassment or painful consequences such as spending sprees, inappropriate sexual activity, speeding, or giving away or wasting money.

- **Clinical Questions.** Have you done or are you now doing things that you may regret or wish you had not done. Are you spending lots of money, becoming sexually involved with people with whom you normally would not be involved and doing things you normally would not do? Will these activities affect your future or result in long-term commitments or problems?
- **Clinical Observations.** The patient, while manic, may brag or talk with enthusiasm about these clearly problematic activities. These actions reflect the poor judgment that often accompanies a manic episode and may be of psychotic proportions.

CASE STUDY: WOMAN WITH MANIA WITH PSYCHOSIS

A 32-year-old woman is brought to the physician by her family because she has experienced a third, similar episode of mania. The patient has, for the past 10 days, been sleeping only 2–4 hours a night, purchased new furniture and drapes for most of the rooms in her house (she works only part-time and cannot afford this), not gone to work, and stated that she wants to set up a bed and breakfast for local farmers to use when they are shopping. She reports that what she is doing will change the national economy, especially for farmers, and will result in an international chain of franchised bed and breakfast facilities. In addition, she has gone to a local bar several times and offered to have intercourse with anyone who is interested. She cannot tell you how many sexual contacts she has had in the back room of the bar but talks of this with pride. She stopped her medication 3 weeks previously because she felt so good she decided she did not need it. During the interview it was very difficult to interrupt the patient's talk about her plans for the house and her sexual needs. She bounced from one topic to another and saw nothing problematic about what she was doing. She refused hospitalization and had to be involuntarily committed. After receiving treatment, which terminated the manic episode, she became very worried about her reputation in the small farming town where she lived and about contracting a sexually transmitted disease. She sought appropriate evaluation and treatment for any diseases she might have contracted and also managed to return over $20,000 worth of merchandise. She did not lose her job.

TREATMENT

Lithium carbonate, which patients respond to 65%–75% of the time, was the only treatment for bipolar disorder for 30 years. Recently, carbamazepine (Tegretol) was officially approved for the treatment of mania. Valproic acid (Depakene) is also used frequently with approximately the same response rate.

Lithium Carbonate

The typical dose of lithium carbonate for adults is 900–1800 mg/d. A blood plasma level of 0.5–1.0 mEq/L is considered a therapeutic dose. This may vary depending on the laboratory that measures the plasma level. Side effects of lithium include fine hand tremors, nausea, and an increased frequency of urination and thirst. This can develop into diabetes insipidus and diarrhea. At toxic levels, confusion, slurred speech, marked gastrointestinal spasms, and, eventually, seizures and death can occur. Lithium should never be used in the first trimester and should be avoided during pregnancy if possible. The physician must watch for the development of hypothyrosis in patients on maintenance therapy.

Carbamazepine

The typical adult dose of carbamazepine is 10–20 mg/kg/d. Patients with blood plasma levels of more than 6–12 mg/L should be monitored for toxicity. No therapeutic level has been established. The side effects of carbamazepine include dizziness, nausea, sedation, dry mouth, headache, and constipation. Pregnant patients should avoid this medication. The physician should check liver function studies prior to treatment and every 6 months thereafter.

Valproic Acid

The normal adult dose of valproic acid is 15–40 mg/kg/d. A blood plasma level of 50–120 mg/L is considered a therapeutic dose. Side effects include mild nausea, diarrhea, and abdominal cramps, but sedation and tremors may occur. Pregnant patients should avoid this medication.

Hypomania

DIAGNOSIS

The criteria for a hypomanic episode are identical to those for a manic episode, except the symptoms are not as severe. Symptoms do not cause significant occupational or social impairment. At times patients report functioning very effectively, more so than usual, finishing tasks quickly, making decisions and carrying them out rapidly, and so on. Psychotic symptoms are absent, and these episodes frequently do not need active treatment.

Cyclothymia

DIAGNOSIS

For at least 2 years, patients must have exhibited numerous episodes of hypomania and numerous periods of depressive symptoms that are not severe enough to be a major depressive episode. During the 2-year period the longest time symptoms have been absent has never been more than 2 months.

TREATMENT

Treatment is symptomatic with the judicious use of antidepressants and mood stabilizers.

CHAPTER 5
Anxiety Disorders

Terry A. Travis, M.D., M.S.Ed.

INTRODUCTION
Definition

Anxiety is a very unpleasant emotion that everyone experiences at certain times. It resembles fear physiologically but differs in that the fear has no rational basis. It ranges from almost instantaneous, overwhelming symptoms with a full autonomic discharge that usually lasts less than 30 minutes **(panic disorder)** to a gradual development over several days of minor to severe feelings of tension **(generalized anxiety disorder).** Anxiety can occur with no stimulus or with a specific stimulus **(phobia or post-traumatic stress disorder [PTSD]).** The patient may experience repetitive unwanted thoughts or perform repetitive acts **(obsessive-compulsive disorder [OCD]).**

Chief Complaint

- "I just cannot relax any more."
- "I suddenly get hot, dizzy, and shaky; my heart pounds; and I feel like I am going to die."
- "I worry that I will pass out in public."
- "I cannot fly because I get so upset."
- "I do not go out and do anything anymore."
- "Sometimes I feel as if I am reliving something that was very dangerous, and I cannot handle it."
- "I keep thinking the same things all the time, over and over."
- "I cannot function because I have to do things over and over."

Differential Diagnosis

The following must be ruled out prior to making a psychiatric diagnosis:

- Cardiac disorders, in particular arrhythmias, mitral valve prolapse, pulmonary emboli, myocardial infarction, and angina
- Endocrine disorders, including hyperthyroidism, hypoglycemia, Cushing's disease, hypoparathyroidism, diabetes, and pheochromocytoma
- Neurologic disorders, including seizures, vertigo, and encephalopathy

- Both prescribed and abused drugs and the symptoms of withdrawal
- Respiratory disorders, such as emphysema
- Asthma, anemia, shock, and head trauma

The physician should take a thorough history and perform a complete physical examination as well as screening laboratory studies to rule out endocrine disorders and toxic or metabolic causes. Depending on the patient's history, an electrocardiogram (ECG), neurologic studies, and other procedures may be indicated. Other psychiatric illnesses such as depression, schizophrenia, and personality disorders are often associated with significant anxiety and must be ruled out prior to initiating treatment.

After an organic cause has been excluded, an algorithm is not needed, as the symptoms and history clearly differentiate between the various anxiety disorders. It is most difficult to separate an anxiety disorder from another mental illness that can occur concurrently. Conversely, the patient may demonstrate many symptoms of anxiety as part of that illness. For example, almost 75% of patients with primary depression have symptoms or complaints of anxiety. It is crucial to distinguish among these disorders to make proper treatment decisions.

SPECIFIC ANXIETY DISORDERS

Panic Attacks

DIAGNOSIS

Panic attacks are relatively common; approximately 35% of the population experiences one every year (Table 5-1). However, panic disorder is relatively rare. It occurs in only 0.7% of the population and is much more prevalent when it occurs with the symptoms of agoraphobia (discussed below).

TABLE 5-1
KEY SIGNS AND SYMPTOMS OF PANIC ATTACKS

Cardiac symptoms of palpitations and a rapid or pounding heart rate	Nausea or abdominal queasiness
Sweating	Feeling dizzy, faint, or lightheaded
Trembling or shaking	Fear of going crazy or losing control
Feelings of shortness of breath (dyspnea) or smothering	Derealization or depersonalization
Feelings of choking	Fear of imminent death
Chest discomfort or pain (often interpreted as a heart attack)	Paresthesias
	Chills or hot flashes

- **Criteria.** The criteria for panic attacks consist of the following key signs and symptoms. At least four of the symptoms listed in Table 5-1 must occur abruptly and peak within 10 minutes for it to be considered a panic attack. It is as if the autonomic nervous system has suddenly turned completely on and is overresponding to any stimulation.
  - **Clinical Questions.** These should be asked in a straightforward manner concerning the symptoms listed above. Often, when patients are asked to describe what they are experiencing or to tell what their symptoms are, they will list several of the key signs and symptoms. When panic attacks occur, the patient will clearly remember the symptoms because they are so striking and frightening. The physician can then ask about other symptoms not mentioned and clarify those described by patient.
  - **Clinical Observations.** The patient can often be observed having a whole or partial panic attack while describing their symptoms or the circumstances of these attacks. The patient sweats and becomes anxious, jittery, and uncomfortable. This is an opportunity to gather details of symptomatology and, of course, to verify the diagnosis. The physician can count the patient's pulse and check for dilated pupils. The mental status of patients experiencing panic attacks is otherwise normal.

Agoraphobia

Agora is latin for *marketplace* and *phobia* means *fear*; hence, the word means fear of the marketplace or public spaces. This type of phobia (see Panic Disorders) is often associated with panic attacks. These patients do not leave home or perform routine activities such as shopping, visiting, driving, and going to appointments because of the fear that they will be unable to leave the situation if panic occurs. The core fear is that of being trapped in public, unable to get away. Anticipatory anxiety, the fear of what may happen in a future situation, is a major component of agoraphobia. Patients never want to have another panic attack and will avoid anything that they feel may stimulate one. Patients realize that the situation is unlikely to actually cause harm and that most people are involved routinely in these activities; however, the fear of another panic attack is sufficient to maintain the phobia. Patients do not like the situation in which they find themselves and are often frustrated, discouraged, and depressed about their condition. They often seek treatment but find that they cannot leave the house for their appointments.

Panic Disorders

These can occur with or without agoraphobia. To meet the diagnostic criteria for a panic disorder, the patient must have experienced recurrent unexpected panic attacks; one isolated attack is not sufficient. The patient also must have experienced at least **one** of the following three symptoms for more than 1 month.

1. The first symptom is persistent worry about the occurrence of more attacks. This is termed **anticipatory anxiety** and can seriously affect the patient's functioning.
2. The second symptom is worrying about the meaning of the attacks. The patient may believe he or she is having a heart attack, losing control, or "going crazy."
3. The third symptom is a change in behavior that significantly affects the patient's daily functioning, such as the development of agoraphobia.

CASE STUDY: WOMAN WITH ANXIETY DISORDER

A 28-year-old woman who supports herself, enjoys work, and has friends and an active social life presented with the chief complaint "I do not know what is happening to me." She described the sudden onset of sweating, rapid heartbeat, feeling lightheaded and dizzy, and feeling as if she could not breathe. She described the time and place where the first episode occurred and related that she had gone to the hospital's emergency room where "they took blood tests, checked my heart with an ECG, and told me I was okay." She was told to seek psychiatric help if any more episodes occurred. At the time she was first seen she had had six to eight attacks, all occurring without an obvious cause in totally different situations. They lasted from 10–40 minutes. She could not determine a stimulus but was able to tell herself, "I know I am not dying, and I will be okay soon." All attacks were very uncomfortable, but the patient was able to continue with what she was doing. Her main concern was, "I feel as if I have lost all control. I worry about when it will happen and when I will feel out of control again." She had no symptoms of depression or other mental disorder, and all physical and laboratory findings were normal. With medication, education, and brief counseling, the symptoms ceased within 2 weeks.

Social Phobias

These are specific phobias about performing in social situations. Patients recognize that the fear of humiliation or embarrassment is irrational and are upset with their inability to function. The fear is persistent and interferes with performing or functioning in social situations. The phobia can be specific, such as public speaking, dancing, or test taking, or can be generalized, such as the fear of being in any social situation. The patient often has anticipatory anxiety and suffers from panic attacks in the feared situation. As a general rule, social phobia causes the patient to withdraw because of a fear of incompetence in the normal give and take of society. He or she may be unable to work or function when any significant interaction with others is needed. Patients may even change their profession to avoid anxiety-provoking situations.

Case Study: Man with Social Phobia

A medical student found himself becoming more and more anxious while making clerkship rounds. He related it specifically to being asked to give a formal presentation, something he had always found difficult. During the clerkship the need to present quickly and in a thorough but well-organized manner overwhelmed the student, and he often was unable to complete a presentation. His write-ups and interviews were well done and accurate, demonstrating that he had the information and ability to organize the data, make an appropriate differential, and create a treatment plan. Medication, exposure therapy, and practice with videotaped feedback helped the student, and after four sessions he needed no further treatment.

Specific Phobias

The criteria for specific phobias are the same as those for social phobias except that the fear is related to a specific object or situation that is not social. Examples include fear of dogs, snakes, spiders, flying, elevators, heights, and injections. These are the most common anxiety disorders and often do not affect the patient's life. The patient is able to provide a clear history that requires little clarification, except to verify that the anxiety or panic occurs only in the specific circumstances described by the patient.

Case Study: Man with Specific Phobia

A 32-year-old healthy male farmer told his physician during an examination that he always faints when stuck with a needle. The physician did not listen and assumed the patient was exaggerating, because the patient was otherwise very healthy, strong, and able to deal with all the physical demands of farming, including delivering animals and giving them shots. The patient fainted before the needle was inserted for a blood sample, fell backward off the examining table, and had to be lifted back onto the table while unconscious. Fortunately, except for some sore, stretched muscles, the patient was unhurt. Treatment consisted of taking blood samples in the future while the patient was lying on the examining table and looking away.

Obsessive-Compulsive Disorder (OCD)

OBSESSIONS

These are recurrent and persistent intrusive thoughts, impulses, or images that the patient recognizes as inappropriate and causing marked anxiety. These thoughts are clearly not related to real-life situations, and the person is unable to control these obsessions by ignoring them or replacing them with other actions or thoughts.

COMPULSIONS

Compulsions are repetitive behaviors the patient performs in an attempt to reduce or prevent the obsession. These thoughts or acts are recognized by the patient as abnormal. They cause marked discomfort, are time consuming, and markedly affect the patient's level of functioning.

Depression must be ruled out, as the negative repetitive thoughts of depression can reach a degree of obsession. Schizophrenia must also be considered because some of the obsessions are severe enough to be considered delusional.

CASE STUDY: WOMAN WITH OBSESSIVE-COMPULSIVE DISORDER

A 24-year-old woman was brought in for therapy by her mother because she was unable to shop or hold a job and was essentially housebound by her compulsions. The patient described rituals that affected all of her activities. She had to constantly think about the minute details of any activity, arrange everything so that nothing would be left to chance, and constantly recheck everything. For example, taking a shower could last 4 hours. She would have to check the soap and towels and arrange them so that if the towel got too wet, she had another one within reach. She also checked the soap to be sure it would last for the duration of the shower. As the patient discussed her compulsions in detail, she became anxious, tense, and aware of the all-consuming and incapacitating aspects of these thoughts and subsequent actions. She described the activities in a clear and logical manner, stating that although they did not make sense to her, unless she performed them she became panicky. She was fully aware and frustrated by her inability to perform the routine activities of daily living because of the compulsions. With medication and counseling she was able to drive a car, shop, and be on time for activities. She was living independently within 6 months.

Post-Traumatic Stress Disorder (PTSD)

DIAGNOSIS

An individual who experiences a trauma "outside the range of usual human experience" and who exhibits a variety of significant symptoms for more than 1 month after the event has occurred may be diagnosed with PTSD. The symptoms involve re-experiencing the trauma with marked interference of normal day-to-day functioning, ongoing arousal symptoms, evidence of emotional numbing, and avoidance of anything referring to the event. Many concentration camp victims have chronic PTSD.

- **Criteria.** When persistently re-experiencing the event, patients have one or more of the following symptoms.
  1. The patient recalls the images, thoughts, and perceptions that occurred during the event.
  2. The patient has recurrent nightmares of the event.
  3. The patient relives the event as a flashback, with or without illusions, hallucinations, and dissociation.
  4. The patient exhibits marked anxiety in response to internal or external cues that bring back the event.
  5. The patient experiences concurrent physiologic responses of fear, panic, or horror to these cues.
- **Criteria.** Arousal symptoms include at least two of the following:
  6. The patient experiences significant sleep problems, irritability and outbursts, decreased concentration, hypervigilance, or a marked startle response.
- **Criteria.** Avoidance and numbing must be present in at least three ways.
  7. Avoiding conversations concerning the event or thinking about it, as well as the loss of memory of important aspects of the event, are examples of avoidance.
  8. The numbing of general feelings is indicated by a decreased interest in almost all activities and feelings of detachment and estrangement from others.
  9. There is a loss of affect and no sense of future.
  - **Clinical Questions.** The patient should be asked the following questions. Are there any events in your life that you keep reliving or thinking about over and over again? Do you have nightmares about this? Are there times when you feel as if you are reliving or re-experiencing the event? Do you feel as if you are back in the event and unaware of your surroundings? What events trigger these feelings? Are you always on guard, watching for something to happen? Do certain things make you jump and feel panicky or scared? What are your feelings on a

day-to-day basis for your family and friends? How do you feel about your future?

- **Clinical Observations.** The patient may look quite anxious and become visibly more distraught when asked to talk about the traumatic event; a panic attack often occurs. The patient may startle easily or jump when outside noises or voices are heard. The patient can suddenly become very angry and hostile when asked about his or her condition and then apologize later.

CASE STUDY: MAN WITH POST-TRAUMATIC STRESS DISORDER

A 45-year-old man came in for treatment of his "alcoholism." The physician taking his history asked if he had served in the military and then asked about his experiences in Vietnam. With obvious pain and anxiety, he described his experiences. He stated spontaneously that he still has nightmares in which he hits his wife or screams until he awakens. He drinks to avoid the dreams. When asked questions to complete the history, he answered that he also felt numb, often feeling distant from his wife and children. He has often felt life was meaningless but has never been suicidal, and he has actively avoided anything that would remind him of Vietnam. During the interview a medical helicopter flew over the building to land at the hospital a block away. He broke into a sweat, jumped out of his chair, looked out the door, and then cowered, shivering, in the corner of the room. When asked, he explained logically and clearly that he had felt as if he were back in Vietnam and about to be killed. Treatment consisted of medication and group therapy through a veterans' support group. Within 6 months he was sleeping without nightmares, received two promotions at work, and was enjoying his family and "making up for lost time loving them." He did not drink after the day he was interviewed.

Generalized Anxiety Disorder

This disorder is generally less severe and causes less dysfunction than the other anxiety disorders. It is *imperative* to rule out panic disorder, as the treatment is different.

DIAGNOSIS

Patients with generalized anxiety disorder have excessive, uncontrolled worries about a variety of activities of everyday life, including work, studies, relationships, and finances. These have to be present more days than not for 6 months or more, and at least three of the following six symptoms must be associated with the worry:

- Feeling restless, keyed up or on edge
- Feeling fatigued
- Mind going blank or having trouble concentrating
- Irritability
- Muscle tension
- Trouble falling or staying asleep

Several of the symptoms listed above are also present in depression. Anxiety is comorbid with depression in up to 40% of patients with depression. It is critical to determine whether depression is present to make the correct recommendations for treatment. Withdrawal from alcohol, antianxiety medication, and other central nervous system (CNS) depressants including street drugs; endocrine disorders, especially hypothyroidism; and excessive intake of caffeine should be ruled out.

CASE STUDY: MAN WITH GENERALIZED ANXIETY DISORDER

A 62-year-old man, a cab driver, has been taking 2–3 mg of alprazolam per day for 15 years. He never takes more, as it sedates him, and he does not like the feeling of higher doses. When he does not take the medication, his symptoms include feeling tense, sleeping poorly, a decreased driving ability, and an inability to finish routine tasks because of constant worries about money, customers, and so on. He is constantly distracted by the tension caused by a general feeling that something "bad" is going to happen. He has no symptoms of depression or panic disorder and has no psychotic thoughts. When he takes the medication, the symptoms abate completely, he is comfortable in his work, and he handles the demands of daily life easily.

TREATMENT

Table 5-2 outlines the basic treatment approach to anxiety disorders and shows that there is overlap in the treatments used.

Behavioral Therapy

Behavioral therapies include desensitization, cognitive behavioral therapy, relaxation training, biofeedback, exposure therapy, and breath control. The patient should be referred to a clinician such as a psychiatrist, psychologist, or professional counselor who is well trained in specific techniques.

Benzodiazepines

The most frequently prescribed drugs in the world, benzodiazepines have significant addictive and withdrawal potential

TABLE 5-2
BASIC TREATMENT APPROACH TO ANXIETY DISORDERS

	Behavior Therapy	Benzo-diazepines	Selective Serotonin-Reuptake Inhibitors	Tricyclic Antidepressants	Beta-Blockers	Buspirone (Buspar)
Panic disorder	X	X	X	X		
Obsessive-compulsive disorder	X		X	X		
Social phobia		X	X		X	
Generalized anxiety disorder		X				X
Post-traumatic stress disorder	X		X	X		
Specific phobia	X					

and should be used cautiously. **Never abruptly stop** these medications, as withdrawal symptoms and seizures have been reported following the discontinuation of even low doses when taken for more than a few weeks. They should be tapered slowly over several weeks. Patients should be told of the abuse potential of these medications and the risks of stopping them abruptly. They should also be warned that benzodiazepines interact strongly with alcohol and can be lethal if combined. Patients should be referred to a psychiatrist if they have not responded to doses of 4-6 mg of alprazolam per day, 40 mg of diazepam per day, 4-6 mg of lorazepam per day, or equivalent doses of other benzodiazepines.

Buspirone

Buspirone, a nonbenzodiazepine, is effective, does not lead to dependency, does not interact with alcohol, and is not a sedative. It must be taken for several weeks to reach maximum effectiveness. In contrast, the effect of benzodiazepines is noted within 1 hour and can be used as needed if the anxiety is intermittent.

Selective Serotonin-Reuptake Inhibitors (SSRIs)

Many SSRIs effectively treat a variety of anxiety disorders. The recommended dosage varies widely, depending on the type of anxiety disorder. Referral to a psychiatrist is indicated for management of treatment with SSRIs.

Tricyclic Antidepressants

Imipramine has been found to be especially effective for panic disorders. Clomipramine is a tricyclic medication that is approved only for the treatment of OCD, not for depression.

Beta-Blockers

Beta-blockers are used on an as needed basis for social phobias such as fear of speaking, test-taking anxiety, and fear of flying. They essentially block some of the distressing symptoms of anxiety such as sweating, rapid heart beat, palpitations, and tremors. Beta-blockers should be used for phobias that occur rarely and in specific situations.

CHAPTER 6
Personality Disorders

Terry A. Travis, M.D., M.S.Ed.

DEFINITION

Every individual develops a characteristic set of behaviors, style of thinking, and emotional responses that define his or her unique personality. This unique combination of personality traits defines how each person copes with life and interacts with others. A patient is diagnosed with a personality disorder when he or she has developed traits with the following characteristics:

- **Longstanding.** Traits have usually manifested by adolescence.
- **Inflexible.** Traits are rigid and are used even when ineffective; they do not change with experience or learning.
- **Maladaptive.** Traits are maladaptive because patients are unable to cope with new and varying situations.
- **Disturbed Relationships.** Personal and work relationships are often disturbed and chaotic or distant.
- **Distress.** These traits result in frequent subjective distress.
- **Ego-syntonic.** Patients see their symptoms as ego-syntonic; the problem is not with them but with life in general and with everyone else.
- **Not Amenable to Treatment.** Patients do not respond to treatment because these traits are ingrained.
- **Exaggerated.** Normal personality traits or groups of traits are exaggerated 2–3 standard deviations from the norm.

CHIEF COMPLAINT

There is no specific complaint that will cue the physician that the patient has a personality disorder. Complaints may focus on psychiatric symptoms of depression, anger, or anxiety; or may focus on the fact that the patient is here only because others (e.g., boss, wife, friends) have told the patient to seek help.

Physicians caring for patients with personality disorders must primarily determine the existence of the disorder, recognize how this affects the physician–patient relationship, and relate to the patient as well as possible while providing quality medical care.

DIFFERENTIAL DIAGNOSIS

The diagnosis of a personality disorder should be considered when a pattern of maladaptive behavior emerges as the history is taken or the physician realizes that his or her response to the patient is unusual for a normal physician–patient relationship. For instance, if you find yourself responding with anger, rejection of the patient, doubting the patient, being over solicitous, or wanting to refuse to treat this patient, your differential diagnosis should include the possibility that the patient has a personality disorder. These nontherapeutic interactions interfere with the provision of medical care.

The physician should focus on obtaining a routine history; there are no clinical questions that can clarify a diagnosis of personality disorder. It often takes several sessions before a psychiatrist confirms such a diagnosis. Time is needed to understand and confirm the pattern of maladaptive behavior and to understand how the patient brings out "abnormal" feelings in the therapist. The diagnosis of a personality disorder *does not* rule in or rule out other mental or physical disorders; thus, there is no differential diagnosis between the existence of a personality disorder and other disorders.

The personality disorder patient affects the physician–patient relationship in the same way everything else in the patient's life is affected (i.e., maladaptively). The physician must approach the patient as any other patient, recognizing the effect the patient's personality is having on the physician–patient interaction. The need for a thorough history and physical is obvious: the physician requires objective data to diagnose a physical or mental disorder.

In the *DSM-IV*, 10 personality disorders are grouped into three clusters. The clusters exist because of similarities of behavior, traits, or symptoms. Specific diagnoses are based on groups of symptoms that often occur together. Following each description of a personality disorder type below is a list of approaches for dealing with negative reactions and providing appropriate care.

CLUSTER A DISORDERS—ODD OR ECCENTRIC GROUP

Paranoid Personality Disorder

Patients with paranoid personality disorder are pervasively suspicious and mistrustful of others, always assuming that people are taking advantage of them, putting them down, or in some way threatening them. They are not delusional or psychotic.

RECOMMENDED PHYSICIAN INTERACTIONS

- Remain very professional.
- Do not expect to be trusted; explain everything in detail and with complete honesty.

- Recognize their oversensitivity to slights and their guarded, suspicious approach to authority figures.
- When they complain or argue, explain and negotiate very openly with them.

Schizoid Personality Disorder

Persons with schizoid personality disorder are loners; they are always detached from any relationship and often are cold and restricted in their responses to others. They get little enjoyment from anything.

RECOMMENDED PHYSICIAN INTERACTIONS

- Respect their aloofness and distance.
- Expect a trusting relationship to be long in developing.
- Expect minimal emotion from the patient.
- Always be scrupulously honest, as patients are exquisitely sensitive to minimization or understatement, often interpreting it as rejection or lack of respect.

Schizotypal Personality Disorder

Persons with schizotypal personality disorder are eccentrics with strange or odd appearance, actions, and thought. They are not psychotic but often have odd beliefs and magical thinking (e.g., believing in signs or omens) and tend to talk in a vague, circumstantial, or stilted manner. They have few friends and are often suspicious of others.

RECOMMENDED PHYSICIAN INTERACTIONS

Similar to interactions with schizoid patients, respect their isolation and uniqueness.

CASE STUDY: WOMAN WITH CLUSTER A DISORDER

The patient was a 47-year-old postal clerk. She entered therapy because she was about to be fired for inadequate performance at work. The patient presented the history in a detached, cold, and unaffected manner. She stated that she thought her work was as good as always, and she did not see any problems. Her mental status examination was normal except for some vagueness in giving details. She had never received nor sought psychiatric treatment previously. She kept appointments punctually. After five or six sessions, the patient started talking about her fascination with numbers. Gradually, in a very circumstantial manner, she detailed how it affected her entire life. She noted patterns between numbers and occurrences in her life. For example, she related the number of cars stopped at each red light on the way to work to magical thinking about how the day or week had been or would be going.

She was friendless except for some people at work with whom she shared lunch. She had had no legal problems and did not use drugs or alcohol. The pattern of numbers she noted influenced with whom she talked and how she planned her daily activities. This had not affected her negatively at work until she became fascinated with the patterns of different sizes and colors of envelopes she handled. Her output decreased, and she became irritable with other employees who interfered with her concentration on observing the number patterns of different types of mail. As a result, she was told she needed psychiatric help to improve her work and keep her job. She had had no previous problems at work. Treatment consisted of listening to her story, obtaining minute details, and helping her identify ways to continue her enjoyment of spontaneous number patterns but delaying the gratification until after work. She would observe and remember the patterns but not slow down until after work to enjoy and meditate on the meaning of what she had observed. After 2 months of practice and support from her therapist, her work productivity returned to normal. She was never depressed or psychotic. She was appropriately concerned about losing her job (which she enjoyed) and was pleased with the help she received in therapy.

CLUSTER B DISORDERS—DRAMATIC, EMOTIONAL, AND ERRATIC GROUP

Antisocial Personality Disorder

Persons with antisocial personality disorder violate the rights of others without conscience. They are unable to control their impulses regardless of the consequences and are unable to postpone immediate gratification. They are insensitive to others, egocentric (they always come first), and demanding, as well as irresponsible, aggressive, impulsive, deceitful, remorseless, and criminal. This disorder occurs much more frequently in men.

Recommended Physician Interactions

- These patients manipulate whenever they can.
- Do nothing that makes you feel uncomfortable or that you would not do for other patients, such as administering extra antianxiety or pain medications or excusing the patient from work when there is nothing wrong with him or her.
- If the patient asks for special favors or wants something done that is not usual practice for good patient care, set firm limits with an appropriate rationale.
- When taking the history, clarify details that the patient presents in a vague or general manner.

Borderline Personality Disorder

People with borderline personality disorder have markedly unstable self-images, moods, and relationships with others. They often cannot be alone for fear of abandonment, have intense but chaotic relationships, are impulsive, have chronic feelings of emptiness, and poor anger control. They are frequently dangerous to themselves, exhibiting recurrent suicidal gestures, attempts, and threats. Some engage in self-injurious behaviors such as burning or cutting themselves. Women are diagnosed more frequently with borderline personality disorder. Brief psychotic episodes can occur under stress, and mood disorders can occur concurrently. There is often a history of sexual abuse during childhood that should be elicited with questions.

RECOMMENDED PHYSICIAN INTERACTIONS

- Treat similarly to antisocial personality disorder.
- The patient may say other physicians or health care providers are good or bad and attempt to get you to take sides for or against others who have provided treatment. This is called *splitting* and can create intense feelings in the physician and staff.
- Set limits and provide quality, conservative treatment.
- The patient should be referred to a psychiatrist for follow-up.

CASE STUDY: WOMAN WITH CLUSTER B DISORDER

The patient was a 35-year-old single woman who always felt empty and isolated from the rest of humanity. She had been sexually abused by numerous family members and was able to talk about this only after 3 years of therapy, when she was able to trust her therapist. She often cut herself when she felt tension building, and she described the cutting as painless and accompanied with a wonderful sense of relief when she saw the blood. She understood that cutting herself was not sufficient cause for hospitalization and would improve after 1–3 days of support in a crisis unit. Occasionally she had all the symptoms of a major depressive disorder that responded only moderately to antidepressants. She never had overtly psychotic episodes but occasionally was fearful of others for no apparent reason and would retreat from all activities and then injure herself. With several years of ongoing psychotherapy and antidepressant medication, she has finished 2 years of college and is working part-time. She now self-mutilates two to four times a year, inflicting superficial cuts that do not require suturing, as was necessary in the past.

Narcissistic Personality Disorder

Patients with narcissistic personality disorder have a grandiose sense of self but are sensitive to all criticism. They often exaggerate what they can do or have done, feel entitled to things, use others, lack empathy, and are arrogant. They love to be admired for their unique and special talents and hate being criticized.

RECOMMENDED PHYSICIAN INTERACTIONS

- These individuals often make people on the treatment team feel angry because patients denigrate the services provided, belittle the intelligence of the caretakers, and expect special treatment.
- Keep calm and remain professional, a difficult but necessary task.
- Diagnoses and recommendations should be explained carefully.

Histrionic Personality Disorder

Persons with histrionic personality disorder are dramatic, seductive, provocative, insincere, and love to be the center of attention. They are emotionally suggestible, their affect changing rapidly depending on the situation.

RECOMMENDED PHYSICIAN INTERACTIONS

- These patients are often very charming and seductive toward physicians of the opposite sex. They have learned how to gain sympathy by being charming or passive.
- Avoid doing anything out of the ordinary for the patient (e.g., ordering higher than usual doses of sleeping medication, making extra, unnecessary rounds to see the patient).
- The professional limits of the physician–patient relationship must be scrupulously maintained.
- Treatment should be conservative, as patients often dramatically exaggerate their symptoms.

CLUSTER C DISORDERS—ANXIOUS AND FEARFUL GROUP

Avoidant Personality Disorder

Patients with avoidant personality disorder are self-critical and have low self-esteem. They are very timid and shy but lonely. They would like to have friends but are so fearful of rejection and criticism that they often avoid social contact, are inhibited in social settings, and are restrained in any relationship.

RECOMMENDED PHYSICIAN INTERACTIONS

- These are often good, compliant patients who seek the physician's acceptance.
- Additionally, these patients are especially sensitive to criticism, and the physician should not say anything that might be construed as a derogatory comment or an insult.

Dependent Personality Disorder

Persons with dependent personality disorder are markedly passive individuals who place their own needs below those on whom they depend. They cannot make routine decisions, want someone else to assume responsibility for their life, never argue, and feel helpless when alone. They always want someone in their life to take care of their needs.

RECOMMENDED PHYSICIAN INTERACTIONS

- When these patients become ill, they feel overwhelmed and helpless and become demanding, complaining, and critical of their care, as if enough cannot be done for them.
- Physicians and staff often get angry and punish the patient by being hostile or telling him or her off.
- The treatment team should decide on setting limits for the patient in response to frequent requests for changes in treatment and frequent complaints.
- The treatment team members should support one another and establish mutually agreed upon and consistent limits.

Obsessive-Compulsive Personality Disorder

Persons with obsessive-compulsive personality disorder are inflexible, live by set rules, keep lists and schedules, and want everything to be perfect and in order. As a result, they often procrastinate, are unable to finish projects, work extremely hard, are unable to throw things away, are overly conscientious, are miserly, and have few friends. They do *not* have obsessive-compulsive disorder. This disorder is seen more commonly in men.

RECOMMENDED PHYSICIAN INTERACTIONS

- It is important that these patients do not feel as if they have lost control of their lives by being placed in the passive role of patient.
- If they feel they have lost control, they will complain about the quality of care they are receiving and be constantly critical.
- Patients are given control by including them in the decision-making process, carefully explaining to them the benefits

and drawbacks of treatment, and giving them flexibility in taking their medication by teaching them the medication's pharmacokinetics. Patients then understand how frequently and why the medication is taken and if an additional dose should be taken if one is missed. When patients feel they are partners in learning about their illness and treatment and can participate in making decisions, they comply with treatment, use their knowledge to maximize their care, and become ideal patients who work well with their physicians in controlling their illness.

CASE STUDY: MAN WITH CLUSTER C DISORDER

The patient was a 42-year-old man who sought therapy on his own volition because, "I cannot do my job like I should, and I am a total failure." He had always been the best salesman in his company (of which he was very proud) and loved his family, but he set all the rules and kept perfect personal financial records. He began doing poorly when his company gave him a promotion, moved him and his family to a new town, and gave him a managerial job with no training or experience. He blamed himself completely for not doing the job perfectly but would not ask for help or advice from his superiors as this, "would show them what a failure I am. I will lose my job, and my family will be destitute." He always came to interviews immaculately dressed in a dark suit and shiny black shoes with every hair combed perfectly in place. He talked about how his teenage sons wanted to grow their hair longer than he let them and did not understand why they did not agree with him about how bad he felt it made them look. His wife described him as a good husband who did everything exactly and in a routine manner. After several sessions he agreed to contact his company regarding problems that he had no idea how to handle. He recognized it was better to do this than to let things deteriorate further. However, since he could not bring himself to make the call personally, he contacted an old friend with whom he had worked in the past. His friend agreed to talk with the company directors and convey the message. The patient could not believe it when the executives of the company apologized for placing him in a position in which he could not succeed and offered to create a special position for him back at the home office. He also received a raise, and all costs of buying a new home and selling his current one were paid. He still felt that he "should have been able to deal with anything, but I will not fail in my new job." Additional counseling as he began his new position allowed him to back off a little from demanding his idea of perfection from his teenage sons. He was amazed when the arguments stopped, his sons no longer wanted to grow their hair long, and they started to care for and show respect for him. His wife reported that he was still incredibly organized but now more able to interrupt what he was doing to spend time with her and the children.

TREATMENT

No good treatment exists for patients suffering from personality disorders. They do not seek treatment until others insist or until they get depressed by how badly life is going. These patients frequently drop out of treatment when their life calms down. Psychotherapy is the best treatment. Establishing a relationship with the patient is often the most difficult and stressful part of treatment for both the patient and therapist. There are no consistent results with a particular therapy, but a variety of cognitive behavioral therapies are currently being used. These appear to produce better results for some patients. They do not focus on emotions but on the styles of thought that result in problems. Patients have to be motivated and willing to do a lot of homework between sessions, as well as attend both individual and group sessions. Medication is helpful only when the patient develops an acute psychosis or a major depressive disorder in response to life stresses. Medication helps with reality testing and mood but not with the basic underlying personality disorder. The team approach often works best. In addition to an individual therapist, crisis beds, a psychiatrist, and other treatment center resources should be available. Patients should be referred to a psychiatrist for evaluation and to a psychotherapist for counseling.

CHAPTER 7
Somatoform, Dissociative, and Factitious Disorders

Terry A. Travis, M.D., M.S.Ed.

INTRODUCTION

Somatoform, dissociative, and factitious disorders are often presented together because all three:

- Appear to have a psychological basis for their signs and symptoms
- Are rule-out diagnoses that are made only when physical or other mental illnesses are excluded
- Require treatment that is nonspecific, and is either symptom-oriented or aimed at uncovering areas of psychological conflict.

SOMATOFORM DISORDERS

The distinguishing feature of somatoform disorders is the presence of symptoms of a physical disorder for which no basis can be found. There must also be evidence that the symptoms meet a psychological need for the patient. These patients rarely are seen by psychiatrists, as they believe their symptoms are physically, not psychologically, based. They comprise a significant portion of patients seen by primary care physicians.

Somatization Disorders

DEFINITION

Somatization disorders are characterized by many of the following factors:

- Patients present with multiple physical symptoms.
- Symptoms, which occur over several years, are unrelated to any known physical disorder.
- Symptoms are clearly beyond any indicated by physical findings.
- Symptoms are severe enough that patients self-medicate, repeatedly seek medical attention, and change life style.
- Patients often see many physicians over time or simultaneously.
- Patient's medical histories are often complicated yet vague or exaggerated.
- Patients have experienced four pain symptoms over the

course of the illness: two gastrointestinal symptoms, one sexual symptom, and one pseudoneurologic symptom.

CHIEF COMPLAINT

- "I have been sickly most of my life."
- "I have lots of things wrong with me."
- "No physician has found out what my problem is. I understand you are good at diagnosis."

DIFFERENTIAL DIAGNOSIS

To exclude common medical and psychiatric illnesses, routine history, physical examination, and basic laboratory studies must be performed. Extensive studies that are minimally indicated or intrusive must be done only after following the patient for several visits and when they are reasonably warranted. This is often a difficult part of decision-making when caring for these patients; the physician does not want to miss something treatable but at the same time does not want to alarm the patient by suggesting that the problem is serious and requires expensive workups and surgery. Avoid iatrogenic complications caused by overtreatment or over-assessment.

CASE STUDY: WOMAN WITH SOMATIZATION DISORDER

The patient is a 42-year-old woman who is seen for recurrent abdominal pain associated with bloating, nausea, and vomiting. She has undergone six abdominal surgeries during the past 24 years with no definitive findings. She has experienced multiple pain symptoms involving several body systems, is rarely able to achieve orgasm because intercourse "is uncomfortable," and often cannot swallow as a result of "throat spasm." She states that no one has found a cause or treatment for her symptoms even though she has seen many physicians and received many different opinions. She has managed to work despite her problems but often runs out of sick days. She is pleasant, cooperative, and eager to give detailed but vague descriptions of her symptoms. There is no evidence of psychosis or a thought disorder; her sensorium is intact, and she appears to be of average intelligence. Her insight is limited, and her judgment is poor, as she often changes physicians, does not follow-up on recommendations, and often self-medicates with a variety of remedies.

TREATMENT

There is no known specific treatment. It is recommended that once a relationship has been established with a patient, the patient should be seen at regular intervals for brief periods of time. Appointments should be made for 15 minutes every 2–4 weeks, and supportive symptomatic treatment given while reassuring the patient that nothing is seriously wrong. New complaints should be heard and noted, followed by an appropriate evaluation. This combination of meeting regularly with and listening carefully to the patient hopefully will minimize unnecessary procedures, evaluations, and treatments. Appointments can often be made further apart over time as the patient accepts the symptoms, learns to live with them, and knows that he or she is receiving care and attention.

Conversion Disorder

DEFINITION

Conversion disorder is the loss or change of a voluntary motor or sensory function that suggests a physical disorder but is better explained as an expression of a psychological need or conflict. The psychological concept of primary and secondary gain is implicit in this definition. The *primary gain* is the repression of an unacceptable drive (usually sexual or aggressive) from the patient's awareness by symbolic expression as a physical symptom. The symptom results in *secondary gain* in the form of help, sympathy, and attention that resolve the conflict.

CHIEF COMPLAINT

- "I went blind yesterday."
- "I cannot move my leg correctly."
- "My hands and feet are numb."

DIFFERENTIAL DIAGNOSIS

The physician must rule out the followinig:

- Any physical, especially neurologic, illness with symptoms similar to conversion disorder
- Dependent or histrionic personality disorders
- Somatization disorder
- Schizophrenia

CASE STUDY: WOMAN WITH CONVERSION DISORDER

The patient, a 38-year-old woman with ongoing financial and family stressors, was being followed for generalized anxiety disorder. She casually reported having gone blind the previous weekend. She was very tired after coming home from work, her 4-month-old son was ill with fever and vomiting, and she had not had time to shop for food for dinner that day. She said, "My son was screaming, my other kids were saying they were hungry, and I was tired; then the phone rang, and I went blind." She reported that she got to the phone by crawling to it by feel. After finishing the conversation on the phone, she then called an ambulance, and she and her children were taken to the local emergency room. She told me, "They did a physical examination, drew blood, and gave me a shot that they said would make things better. My sight came back gradually over the next hour, and I have been fine since then. I do not know what was in the shot." She presented this history in a matter-of-fact way without marked emotion, as if she was describing having a headache. She never had another episode of conversion symptoms. The patient's *primary gain* was alleviation of the anger she felt in her situation that might have led to child abuse. The *secondary gain* was the resolution of her immediate stress by being taken to the hospital, where the children were fed and watched until she was able to assume her usual role of single parent and provider.

TREATMENT

The primary treatment is support and alleviation of the stressors that precipitated the conversion. Individual and group therapies are often helpful. Other people in the patient's life, who may be providing ongoing secondary gain in response to the patient's symptom, should be involved in the therapy to break the cycle of supporting the symptom. Hypnosis or an amobarbital interview is helpful occasionally for rapid relief but seldom necessary, and referral to a psychiatrist is appropriate when considering this treatment modality. Medication does not help. For the woman in the case study above, her improvement was a nonspecific response to the attention received, the relief of her stressors, and her giving credit to the shot for "curing" her.

Somatoform Pain Disorder

DEFINITION

Somatoform pain disorder is considered a conversion disorder with only one symptom, pain. Psychological factors are important but are not necessary for diagnosis. The preoccupation is clearly excessive considering the physical and laboratory findings, and possible physical and psychiatric disorders must be ruled out.

CHIEF COMPLAINT

- "I have this pain in my head, arm, penis, rectum, abdomen (any location) that will not go away. No one has been able to find the cause and provide relief."

DIFFERENTIAL DIAGNOSIS

The physician must exclude all physical and mental disorders that cause symptoms of pain in that area.

Case Study: Man with Somatoform Pain Disorder

The patient was a 68-year-old man who developed a constant, aching pain in his penis 6 years ago. The pain started 3 months after his wife died from disseminated breast cancer. The cancer was discovered 6 months before she died. The patient's pain did not vary with urination, and all urogenital and neurologic studies were normal. The pain was not relieved by pain medication, including narcotics and antidepressants, or electroconvulsive therapy (ECT). The patient has been in supportive counseling, has visited several pain clinics, and has learned skills to cope with the pain. Currently he takes no medication, except occasionally something to help him sleep.

Treatment

Patients with somatoform pain disorder are given the following:

- A trial of an antidepressant medication
- Referral to a pain clinic for a multidisciplinary approach to pain management
- Support groups and behavioral techniques such as relaxation, medication, and self-hypnosis. Opiates, sedatives, and antianxiety medications should *not* be administered. The goal is to reduce pain-related behavior and resume normal daily activities.

Hypochondriasis

Definition

Hypochondriasis is best characterized by the following:

- Fear of having or the belief that one has a serious physical illness, often based on real signs, symptoms, or sensations
- Fear that is not relieved when the physical examination and laboratory and investigative procedures are found to be normal
- A duration of symptoms for 6 months or more

Chief Complaint

- "I know I am dying from cancer."
- "I am not as coordinated as I used to be, and I am sure I have Lou Gehrig's disease."
- "My heart is failing because of the way it beats."

Differential Diagnosis

The physician must consider and exclude all physical and mental disorders.

Case Study: Woman with Hypochondriasis

The patient is a 38-year-old woman who currently lives with her mother. She works irregularly because she always feels tired, weak, and "just not well." For the past 2 years she feels that a chronic liver infection has caused the fatigue, occasional aches, loss of energy, and a dull ache throughout her abdomen. Repeated liver function studies have revealed no abnormalities. Magnetic resonance imaging (MRI) and sonography also have revealed no abnormalities. She is taking vitamin supplements and other natural products from a local health food store but is not taking prescribed medication. She has requested an evaluation.

Treatment

- Psychotherapy and psychotropic medications do not help these patients.
- Unnecessary procedures should be avoided.
- The physician should set fixed appointments at regular intervals.
- The physician should maintain an accepting and supportive attitude toward the patient.

DISSOCIATIVE DISORDERS

Dissociative disorders rarely occur. This group of psychiatric disorders involves the sudden loss or disruption of memory, identity, or behavior.

Dissociative Amnesia

Dissociative amnesia is the sudden onset of memory loss following a traumatic experience.

Chief Complaint

- "I cannot remember anything that happened the 3 days before coming to the hospital."
- "I do not remember anything about myself."

Differential Diagnosis

Physicians must consider and exclude the following:

- Dementia
- Alcoholic or substance-induced blackouts
- Alcohol amnestic syndrome (Korsakoff's syndrome)
- Postconcussion amnesia
- Malingering
- Postictal confusion

CASE STUDY: WOMAN WITH DISSOCIATIVE AMNESIA

A 25-year-old woman was admitted to the hospital 1 week after her house burned to the ground. Her two children died in the fire, and she was the only survivor. She had no memory of this event. She had no previous psychiatric history, and all findings on the physical examination and laboratory studies were normal. She re-lived the experience during an amobarbital interview and re-sponded well to supportive and grief therapy. She was discharged 3 days after being hospitalized and has been attending a support group for individuals who have lost their children.

TREATMENT

Care should focus on the following:

- Removing the stressor from the patient's life
- An amobarbital interview or hypnosis initially
- Supportive psychotherapy as follow-up

Dissociative Identity Disorder (Multiple Personality Disorder)

DEFINITION

Multiple personality disorder is the presence of two or more distinct identities in which at least two of these identities recur-rently take control of the person's behavior. The therapist may observe marked changes in personality styles, presentation, and clothes at different appointments.

CHIEF COMPLAINT

- "I lose periods of time when I do not know what I have done."
- "I am told by friends that I do things and behave differently at times."

DIFFERENTIAL DIAGNOSIS

The physician must exclude the following:

- Other psychiatric disorders
- Complex partial seizures
- Substance-abuse disorders

CASE STUDY: WOMAN WITH MULTIPLE PERSONALITY DISORDER

The patient was a 27-year-old certified public accountant. She first complained of suicidal preoccupation, an inability to relate to people, and intermittent auditory hallucinations. The patient had held her current position after graduation from college and was about to be made a partner in the firm. She appeared markedly depressed with notable psychomotor slowing. She responded poorly to antidepressants and participated minimally in counseling. The therapist called the patient at work one day to reschedule an appointment and was astounded to hear the patient speaking in a different voice and style, fully animated and assertive. The patient told the therapist that "she" would come to the next appointment and tell her what was going on. At the next appointment the patient was dressed differently than at previous appointments, showed no evidence of depression, and presented herself as an assertive professional. The patient then told the therapist about her three different personalities, stating that only one had come to the clinic previously. She related a story of sexual abuse involving intercourse with her father that started when she was 12 years of age and had continued to the present. She talked about homicidal plans and wishes and stated that the depressed personality took over whenever she was with her parents. Her mother denied that anything wrong was happening, and her father threatened to harm her if she told anyone about their ongoing sexual relationship. She functioned effectively at work as the professional person that knew nothing about the depressed person or the one presenting this new information. Counseling continued, and all medication was stopped. Gradually, over the next 2 years, the patient began reducing contact with her parents and refusing to have intercourse with her father.

TREATMENT

Long-term psychotherapy is necessary, and an appropriate referral should be made. Hospitalization is needed during periods of crisis such as suicidal or homicidal ideation or self-injury.

Dissociative Fugue

DEFINITION

A dissociative fugue is the loss of memory of one's past combined with travel away from one's home or place of work and the assumption of a new identity.

CHIEF COMPLAINT

- "I found myself working at a job and living at a place that I had never been before."

DIFFERENTIAL DIAGNOSIS

Disorders should be excluded the same way as in dissociative amnesia and dissociative identity disorder.

Case Study: Man with Dissociative Fugue

The patient was a 25-year-old married sales clerk with one daughter. A month after he disappeared from work and home, he found himself working in a town at a gas station more than 1500 miles from home. He remembered nothing about getting there, obtaining the job, or where he lived while he was there. He did remember that his wife had told him about an extramarital affair she had had for 2 years and that she had asked for a divorce. He returned home and began counseling with his wife.

Treatment

Patients with dissociative fugue should be treated with supportive psychotherapy.

Depersonalization Disorder

Definition

Depersonalization disorder consists of persistent or recurrent feelings of detachment from one's surroundings (derealization) or from one's self (depersonalization) that cause significant distress.

Chief Complaint

- "I find myself tuning out at work and feeling that I am not there but just watching a movie."
- "Sometimes when driving I feel that I am playing a game on the computer, that nothing is real. It really frightens me and I have to pull over and stop."

Differential Diagnosis

The physician needs to exclude the following:

- Side effects of medications or substances.
- Central nervous system diseases such as tumor or epilepsy
- Other mental disorders

Case Study: Man with Depersonalization Disorder

The patient was a 52-year-old man who came for counseling because of "spells where everything looks strange." These spells started after his company was sold and many of his peers were laid off. He described going to committee meetings and suddenly feeling as if he was watching from outside of himself; the surroundings appeared smaller than normal, voices were high and distant, and he was no longer himself but an observer seeing all of this for the first time. He had no symptoms of anxiety or psychosis and was appropriately concerned about these episodes, mostly because often he would not participate in the meeting or answer questions when these spells occurred. His superiors had raised concerns about his performance and the patient's interest in his job. Supportive therapy and talking about his fears and anger resolved his symptoms within 3 weeks.

Treatment

Psychotherapy is the treatment of choice for persons with depersonalization disorder.

FACTITIOUS DISORDERS

Definition

The patient simulates the signs and symptoms of a physical or mental disorder to assume the role of a sick person. No external incentives exist for assuming the role of a sick person, such as in the case of malingering, where a legal settlement may result in a large financial gain or the patient is avoiding the legal responsibility of going to jail or paying debts.

Factitious Disorder with Physical Symptoms (Munchausen Syndrome)

Most patients with this disorder have intermittent, mild illnesses that often occur in response to specific stress. They have a stable family and occupation. These patients are often willing to consider psychiatric intervention as part of their treatment. Munchausen syndrome is a particularly severe subset of factitious disorders. This syndrome is characterized by sociopathic traits, marked resistance to treatment, multiple hospitalizations covering an ever-widening area, and threatening behavior on confrontation.

Chief Complaint

Patients may present with any physical symptom.

Differential Diagnosis

The physician must therefore exclude all physical illnesses.

Case Study: Woman with Munchausen Syndrome

The patient was a 42-year-old woman who was admitted because of lesions infected with *Staphylococcus* on her back and legs. After a full workup the staff became suspicious, as new lesions appeared despite antibiotic therapy. They discovered by accidental observation that the patient was inserting her finger in her rectum and then scratching herself to put feces into the scratch. She infected her back by using a back scratcher that was contaminated with her own feces. When confronted with this, she denied this behavior and became more demanding in her requests. When a consulting psychiatrist entered the room and introduced himself as such, the patient began screaming that she was not crazy, jumped out of bed, began packing her clothes, and wanted to leave. She refused to talk with the psychiatrist and started to walk out of the room and the hospital. Security was called, and the patient sat in her room yelling that she was not crazy and that she would sue. She was allowed to sign out against medical advice when the attending psychiatrist agreed that she could not be committed, as she did not present an immediate danger to herself or others. She left and was never heard from again. Three days later, records arrived from another hospital. She had signed permission for them to be sent. The records detailed an identical history and also reported that she had been to at least 30 different hospitals within the area and repeated the same behavior at each place.

TREATMENT

Most patients improve with supportive, insight-oriented psychotherapy and should be referred for this treatment. Those with full-blown Munchausen syndrome are not amenable to treatment.

CHAPTER 8
Adjustment Disorders

Terry A. Travis, M.D., M.S.Ed.

DEFINITION

An adjustment disorder must meet several criteria before diagnosis.

- The behavioral or emotional symptoms must be in response to an *identifiable stressor*.
- The symptoms must occur *within 3 months* of the onset of the stressor.
- The symptoms cannot persist longer than *6 months after* the stressor has ended. If the disturbance lasts *less* than 6 months, it is specified as *acute*. If the disturbance lasts *more* than 6 months, it is considered *chronic*.
- The symptoms are clinically important because they are beyond that normally expected.
- The symptoms cause *significant impairment* in social, academic, or occupational functioning.
- The symptoms do not meet the criteria for an Axis I disorder and are not part of an existing Axis I or Axis II disorder.

CHIEF COMPLAINT

- "I have not been able to do anything well since I did not get the raise I expected."
- "I am all keyed up, cannot focus and do what I want, feel tired but cannot get to sleep since being laid off due to my company downsizing."
- "Since my wife started divorce proceedings, I have been drinking too much, have received two tickets for speeding, and I have maxed out my credit card."

DIFFERENTIAL DIAGNOSIS

- All mental disorders must be considered and ruled out. The diagnosis of adjustment disorder is made by the process of exclusion.
- The sequential relationship of symptoms to the stressor must be established.
- The duration and severity of the stressor must be evaluated.
- The patient's total personality style must be assessed to exclude a personality disorder.

SPECIFIC DISORDERS

The diagnosis is made based on the type of symptoms that predominate.

- **With depressed mood,** crying, sadness, and feelings of helplessness and hopelessness predominate.
- **With anxiety,** tenseness, nervousness, worry, and feeling on edge are predominate.
- **With mixed anxiety and depressed mood,** a combination of these symptoms occurs.
- **With disturbance of conduct,** behavior that violates the rights of others and breaks the norms and rules of society predominate. Truancy, vandalism, reckless driving, overcharging credit cards, fighting, and skipping work are seen.
- **With mixed disturbance of emotions and conduct,** there are marked emotional and behavioral symptoms.

A normal grief reaction after the death of a loved one is not diagnosed as an adjustment disorder with depressed mood. However, if symptoms of a major depressive disorder exist 2 months after the loss, that diagnosis is appropriate.

TREATMENT

Individual psychotherapy or crisis intervention is the primary treatment. Support and self-help groups are beneficial when they relate directly to the stressor.

Medication is *not* indicated. However, many clinicians do treat the patient symptomatically for a brief time until coping skills are re-established and normal day-to-day functioning returns. If sleeping medication or antianxiety medication is used, it should be time limited, and the patient should be reassessed as often as every 2 weeks. Antidepressant medication is not recommended because of the 2–4 week time to onset of effectiveness. Most patients with adjustment disorder begin to function well within that time. Medication may mask the underlying reason the patient has reacted so strongly to the stressor. Additionally, medication may decrease the patient's motivation to change and develop new and more mature coping skills to adapt to life stresses. The patient may also develop a psychologic or physical dependence on the medication.

CHAPTER 9
Developmental Disorders/ Mental Retardation

Robert J. Pary, M.D.

DEFINITION

Mental retardation is *any* condition that begins before 18 years of age that is characterized by:

- An IQ of 70 or less
- Impairments in at least two of the following areas of adaptive functioning:

  - Communication
  - Self-care
  - Home living
  - Social/interpersonal skills
  - Use of community resources

  - Functional academic skills
  - Self-direction
  - Work
  - Leisure
  - Health
  - Safety

CHIEF COMPLAINT

Patients with mild or moderate retardation present with chief complaints comparable to those in the general population. Individuals with mild mental retardation often are able to verbalize their feelings and describe their symptoms. The physician should take a complete medical history, the same as with any patient. The complaints may be presented in a concrete fashion without elaboration. When the physician asks a question while taking the history, the patient may nod his or her head in agreement. Make sure the patient understands the words or phrases being used. Ask the same question twice but switch the order of the response. First ask, "Are you happy or sad?" then ask, "Are you sad or happy?" If the patient does not understand the question, the last choice is often selected.

A similar problem occurs when individuals use words or phrases they do not understand. For example, patients may say they have ulcers when they mean hemorrhoids, or hysterectomy when they mean appendectomy.

Do not assume that persons with mental retardation understand time concepts. Asking a person if he or she has had trouble sleeping for the past 2 weeks is meaningless if the patient does not know the length of a week.

Collateral sources of information are helpful, even with verbal individuals who have mild mental retardation. Confidentiality must be respected. However, in most instances the individual (or the guardian, if the person is judged incompetent) readily grants permission to contact others who are knowledgeable about the patient.

For individuals with more severe levels of mental retardation, the chief complaint is often made by the caretaker, who notes changes in the patient's function or behavior. The patient's performance of usual activities of daily living may be altered or impaired, or the onset of new behaviors may be seen, such as withdrawal, uncooperativeness, physical aggression toward others, or self-injurious behavior (SIB).

DIFFERENTIAL DIAGNOSIS

The evaluation must consider and exclude possible psychiatric illnesses and medical problems. Occasionally, individuals report or signal that they are in pain. Alternatively, they may rub the part of the body that is causing them discomfort. The first clue to an undiagnosed medical condition may be the onset of or an increase in maladaptive behavior such as physical aggression or SIB. It is impossible to discuss every potential medical cause; however, frequently occurring conditions include:

- Middle ear infections
- Migraine headaches
- Abscessed teeth
- Cellulitis
- Infections around foreign body insertion sites (e.g., string in the nose or plastic pieces in the urethra)
- Respiratory infections
- Urinary tract infections
- Kidney stones
- Partial bowel obstruction from foreign body ingestion
- Undiagnosed fractures

SPECIFIC DISORDERS

Individuals with developmental disabilities can suffer from any of the mental illnesses that occur in the general population, such as major depression, mania, and schizophrenia. Between one-fifth and one-third of all individuals with mental retardation are "dually diagnosed" with mental illness and mental retardation. The two cases presented below discuss the issues of diagnosis, treatment, and management.

CASE STUDY: DEPRESSION IN A MAN WITH MILD RETARDATION

Mr. A. was a 35-year-old man with mild mental retardation who lived alone in an apartment. He complained about wanting to kill himself at work. During the course of the interview, he complained of depressed mood, early morning awakening, trouble concentrating, and recurrent thoughts of suicide. These symptoms had been present for at least 6 months. His physician did not ask, and Mr. A. did not reveal, that he drank 18–24 beers each weekend. Later, it was determined that his supervisor at work suspected that Mr. A. had a drinking problem, but she did not contact the clinic and the physician did not call her. Mr. A. had significant psychomotor agitation. He promised his physician that he would not act on his suicidal thoughts before contacting the clinic or the emergency room. Satisfied that Mr. A. was not at acute risk of harming himself, the patient was placed on selective serotonin-reuptake inhibitors (SSRIs), and Mr. A. was scheduled to return in 21 days. Mr. A.'s physician started him on paroxetine, 20 mg/d. Mr. A. was no better 3 weeks later. His physician increased the dose of paroxetine to 40 mg/d. Suicidal ideation was still present. Two months after the initial interview, Mr. A. was frustrated that he was not doing better. He remembered that the physician said it could take the medicine a couple of months to work. It had been 2 months, and he still felt depressed, although less than when he started the paroxetine. He lost his follow-up appointment card (9 weeks after the initial evaluation) and ran out of paroxetine. Mr. A. had expected to be free from depression at this point. He did not call the clinic to find out the date of his next appointment. Gradually, the depression worsened, and his drinking increased. Three months after the initial interview, Mr. A. overdosed on 20 aspirin and a fifth of vodka.

This case study illustrates four issues: First, although the diagnosis of major depression is straightforward, the physician failed to inquire about substance abuse while taking the general medical history. Persons with mild forms of mental retardation who live in unsupervised apartments are as susceptible as the general population to substance abuse.

Second, the physician did not use collateral sources of information, such as the supervisor at work.

Third, although Mr. A. knew he would not feel better immediately, the physician said he would return to his normal mood in a couple of months. Mr. A. interpreted his physician's statement concretely. When 2 months had passed and Mr. A. still felt depressed, he lost confidence in the medication. Additionally, Mr. A. did not recognize that his depression had improved. Instead, he viewed his response as all or nothing. The physician needs to be aware of the patient's potential for concrete thought. This may be difficult for the physician to recognize, because the patient often nods his head in agreement with whatever the physician says.

Fourth, many individuals with mild mental retardation who are not in a formally supervised setting "fall through the cracks" unless active outreach is present. All persons involved in the patient's care should be told the recommendations to help keep track of appointments and understand the nuances of the information the physician has provided.

CASE STUDY: SIB IN A WOMAN WITH SEVERE MENTAL RETARDATION AND DOWN SYNDROME

Ms. B. was a 22-year-old woman with severe mental retardation and Down syndrome who was brought to the clinic by her case manager. The case manager provided the following information. Ms. B. lived at home and was on a waiting list for a supervised setting. For the past year, her mother's rheumatoid arthritis and migraines had worsened, and she was unable to care for her. Furthermore, Ms. B.'s younger sister went away to college 7 months ago. For the past 6 months, Ms. B. had been hitting her ears with her fist and scratching her temples. This resulted in several abrasions and lacerations. The wounds looked reddened and swollen, and had an exudate. When Ms. B. was not hitting herself, she was often lethargic. She had lost 15 lbs and was sleeping poorly. Family history revealed a depressed father, who was currently on medical leave because of major depression. He had been staying in his bedroom with the drapes pulled during much of the day. Ms. B.'s medical history was significant for frequent ear infections.

The differential diagnosis for her SIB is extensive. Medical conditions should be excluded, such as otitis media, cellulitis, migraine headaches, and thyroid disease (those with Down syndrome are at increased risk). Psychiatric disorders to consider include major depression.

Psychosocial issues that directly affect the patient include her mother's rheumatoid arthritis that interferes with her availability to Ms. B., her sister's move to college, and her father's withdrawal because of depression. Furthermore, because of her age (22 years), Ms. B. may have recently left school and may be staying home all day rather than attending day training. If Ms. B. is home all day, increased tension may result between her and her father or mother, because her mother's rheumatoid arthritis is worsening and other psychosocial stresses are affecting her.

Finally, the SIB may be a form of communication. Determine if any tasks or requests are associated with the self-injury. For example, is the SIB worse when Ms. B. is asked to get out of bed and dress for breakfast? Is the SIB worse when her father or mother leaves the home? Does her family ignore Ms. B. except when she injures herself?

Perhaps the biggest mistake is to assume that the patient cannot be affected by psychosocial issues because she is severely mentally retarded. Psychosocial stresses can upset persons at all levels of mental retardation. Treatment decisions for Ms. B. are the same as for anyone in the general population. Consider all of the possibilities, systematically treat the most likely one first, and continue down the list until Ms. B. responds to therapy.

TREATMENT

For persons with milder forms of mental retardation and clear psychiatric diagnoses, treatment follows the usual guidelines for the general population. Treatment is divided into four parts: patient education, caretaker instructions, nonpharmacologic treatment, and pharmacologic treatment.

Patient Education (If Applicable)

Inform the individual about his or her illness and treatment; do not avoid or ignore the patient just because he or she is mentally retarded. Of equal importance, do not assume that patients "get it" when they nod their heads in agreement. Check again that the person not only can repeat the instructions but also understands their meaning. For some individuals, their receptive language skills are much better than their expressive use of language. An individual's lack of language does not necessarily mean that he or she cannot understand simple information.

Caretaker Instructions (If Applicable)

Caretaker education is potentially more complicated, as the educational background varies widely among caretakers, and turnover occurs frequently. Staff who accompanies the patient may not have adequate contact with the patient or the direct care staff. For all of the above reasons, written communication often is best. For complicated cases involving numerous staff involved in the patient's work and living arrangements, one page of concrete steps outlining how the agency should respond to the patient's aggression or SIB is invaluable. A copy should be kept in the front of the chart as well.

Nonpharmacologic Treatment

For persons in group homes or supervised settings, or when the person is living with family, consider nonpharmacologic treatments such as reinforcing positive behavior. In some settings, praise is not dispensed often enough. Observing how staff or family interact with the patient in the waiting room or during the interview may indicate whether positive reinforcement is freely used. Family and staff should be given guidance and specific suggestions.

When physical aggression is the focus, consider anger management for those individuals with moderate or mild mental retardation who are able to solve problems.

It is important to recognize that individual choice is a part of treatment. For example, some individuals with mental retardation are required to attend a specific day program or have certain room-mates. This works well if the person likes the work or the room-mates, but it can be disastrous when a major conflict occurs. For example, an individual with mild mental retardation and blindness became severely self-injurious and aggressive toward others by flail-ing out with his cane. He had recently moved to a two-person apartment with a roommate. Everyone working with this patient felt good that he no longer lived in an institution or a large 15-bed group home. After several months, the individual said that he hated where he lived because his roommate often moved the furniture and the stereo. This made his mobility, or even finding the stereo, quite difficult. He felt that no one would listen to him because everyone had told him what a great accomplishment it was to move from an institution, to a 15-bed home, and finally to an apartment. The solution was not a behavior program or medication but a change in his living arrangement.

Pharmacologic Treatment

This chapter does not cover all pharmacologic treatments. In-stead, it focuses on the differences between treating develop-mentally disabled patients and treating patients in the general population.

Perhaps the biggest difference is that medication decisions should be "data-driven," meaning that, whenever possible, rating scales or data collected by caretakers over time should strongly influence these decisions. Data are emphasized to avoid irrational treatment decisions based more on emotion than facts. For exam-ple, if an informant focuses on a recent incident of aggression, it is more important to use the overall aggression rate for the past 12 months in any decision concerning medication changes. If the major focus is on last incident, the temptation is to increase or change the medication. In the above scenario, if the aggression rate is 50% lower since the last visit and 90% lower in the last year, no change in dose or medication is needed.

The second difference, particularly if the patient has previously been in an institution, is that all medication the patient is taking should be assessed to determine if any can be reduced or discon-tinued. Persons with mental retardation are some of the most medicated members of society. The most frequently prescribed psychotropics are neuroleptics, often used to treat psychosis. Psy-choses, however, have been overdiagnosed in this group of patients. For example, a physician may mistake the patient's self-talk for hallucinations. It is important to watch for and detect side effects because of the risk of akathisia or tardive dyskinesia.

CHAPTER 10
Substance-related Disorders

Ronald W. Kanwischer, M.A., C.A.D.C.

DEFINITION

A substance-related disorder is a maladaptive relationship with alcohol or other drugs. Problems related to substance use are divided into two categories, substance use disorders and substance-induced disorders. The substance use disorders are substance abuse and substance dependence.

Substance Use Disorders

Substance abuse is a maladaptive, recurrent pattern of drug or alcohol use that results in repeated negative consequences for the user. The person is willing to continue using the substance despite repeated problems. For example, a young man uses cannabis on a weekly basis. Although aware that his grades have dropped because he is often intoxicated during school, he continues to use the drug. He is willing to sacrifice good grades for the benefits he believes he gets from cannabis. This pattern of use and consequences must occur within a 12-month period and must not meet the criteria for the more severe substance dependence disorder.

Substance dependence disorder is typified by inconsistent and impaired control over when and how much of the substance is used, resulting in significant consequences. This characteristic pattern of compulsive use often leads to the development of tolerance and withdrawal. Neither is essential nor sufficient by itself to establish the diagnosis. The substance use becomes so important that it begins to define the person's life style, as indicated by their priorities, activities, and companions.

Substance-induced Disorders

The substance-induced disorders cause a variety of symptoms that may mimic other medical, mental, and neurologic conditions. Establishing a differential diagnosis is difficult. However, the important distinction to make is that the symptoms are *best* explained by the direct effect of a substance. Look for evidence of recent use of a substance (including illicit, prescription, or over-the-counter preparations), intoxication, or withdrawal. These disorders are: substance intoxication, substance withdrawal, substance-induced delirium, substance-induced persisting dementia, substance-induced persisting amnestic disorder, substance-induced psychotic disorder, substance-induced mood disorder, substance-induced anxiety disorder, substance-induced sexual dysfunction, and substance-induced sleep disorder. The most commonly encountered disorders are **substance intoxication** and **substance withdrawal.**

CHIEF COMPLAINT

- "My spouse has threatened to leave me if my drinking continues. I am not sure I can stop on my own."
- "I have battled the booze for years."
- "I have just gotten my second driving under the influence (DUI) citation."
- "Every time I try to stop using heroin, I get shaky and sick."
- "I have failed a urine test at work, so now I must have a substance abuse evaluation."
- "My cardiologist says that if I do not quit smoking, I will have another heart attack."

DIFFERENTIAL DIAGNOSIS

Many behaviors suggest drug or alcohol abuse. Approximately 80% of adult Americans use alcohol at some time during their lives. Nonpathologic use of substances is common in the United States, particularly alcohol, prescription drugs, and over-the-counter preparations. Substance abuse or dependence is distinguished from nonpathologic use by the presence of substance-related problems, compulsive use, tolerance, and withdrawal.

Screening and Evaluation

Many paper and pencil tests are used to assist in the screening and evaluation of substance use disorders. The most effective have a sensitivity and specificity of over 90%. One of the more useful screening questionnaires for detecting alcohol dependence is an interview mnemonic device termed the **CAGE.**[1]

Cut down: "Have you ever considered cutting down or stopping your alcohol use?"

Annoyed: "Have you ever felt annoyed or irritated if someone criticized your drinking?"

Guilt: "Have you ever felt guilty about your drinking or things you did while intoxicated?"

Eye-opener: "Have you ever used alcohol in the morning to chase away a hangover or steady your nerves?"

---

[1] Ewing JA: Detecting alcoholism: the CAGE questionaire. *JAMA* 252:1905–1907, 1984.

Two or three positive responses suggest an alcohol problem, and four positive responses are pathognomonic for alcohol dependence. The CAGE can be adapted to screen for drug dependence without loss of sensitivity or specificity by simply including the word "drugs" in the four questions. This is then termed the **CAGE-AID.**

A careful and structured interview should then be conducted (including significant others if possible). The interview encompasses a review of the *Diagnostic and Statistical Manual of Mental Disorders*, 4th ed. (*DSM-IV*) criteria (see *clinical questions*), including:

- Historical and current information related to the quantity, frequency, and type of substances used
- Method of administration
- Preoccupation with and efforts to control use
- Concern expressed by the patient or others
- Consequences of the substances used in the six basic domains (familial, legal, social, occupational or financial, medical, psychologic functioning)
- Family history
- Past treatments and response
- Recovery environment (supportive or otherwise)
- Motivation to change
- Level of insight

In the *DSM-IV*, less emphasis is placed on tolerance and withdrawal (the older and classic concept of addiction), and more emphasis is placed on the consequences of a patient's use and impairment of control. Therefore, the physician should focus less on the quantity and frequency of use, which can be distorted intentionally or by poor memory, and more on the problems caused by the substance use. Since the substance use disorders are diagnosed by history, it is very important that the physician gathers accurate data. Patients may distort their histories for many reasons, but this can be minimized in several ways. Enter into the interview with the understanding that the patient is *suffering* from their substance use problem, even if it seems to be of their own doing. This helps to establish a good rapport with the patient. They will be watching your reaction to their answers very closely, looking for signs of disapproval or judgment. (Addicts see that all the time.)

- Make sure that the patient is not intoxicated or in the middle of uncontrolled withdrawal during the interview. Use a structured interview based upon the *DSM-IV* criteria, and use instruments with good reliability and validity.
- Make sure that the patient has no obvious reason for distort-

ing the information. For example, an adolescent may be worried that you will tell his or her parents, a young mother who is in trouble with child welfare for using substances may risk losing her child, or a person on parole and under court order to remain sober may fear being sent back to prison.

- Let the patient know that you will check several sources of information, such as old records, laboratory findings, and collaterals.
- Assure them that the information is confidential, unless other circumstances or arrangements are made.

A complete medical history should be taken, and a physical examination and laboratory studies should be completed. Laboratory studies are often inconclusive and show great variability. They should be used only in conjunction with other sources of information. Currently, no laboratory marker has proven to measure excessive alcohol use consistently and reliably. γ-Glutamyltransferase (GGT) is increased in more than half of patients with alcohol problems and in approximately 80% of patients with alcoholic liver dysfunction. Aspartate transaminase (AST) is increased in approximately 50% of patients with alcohol dependence. A decreased white blood cell (WBC) count and increased mean corpuscular volume (MCV) are common. Uric acid, triglyceride, and urea levels also may be increased.

SPECIFIC DISORDERS

Substance-induced Disorders

Many medical conditions mimic substance-induced disorders, particularly intoxication and withdrawal (e.g., fluctuating consciousness, slurred speech, incoordination, unsteady gait).

- If a symptom appears while under the influence of a substance, then gradually disappears as the person sobers, it can be attributed to *intoxication*.
- If a symptom appears after stopping or reducing the use of a substance, it is likely to be caused by *withdrawal*.

DIAGNOSIS OF SUBSTANCE ABUSE

The person must have experienced *one or more* of the following symptoms within a *12-month period* to meet the criteria for substance abuse.

1. Criterion. Recurrent substance use resulting in a failure to fulfill major obligations at work, school, or home.

- **Clinical Questions.** Do you ever use drugs (or alcohol) while at school or work? Have you ever been high (or drunk) at school or work? Do you ever miss school or work because you are high (or drunk or recovering from a hangover)? Have your grades (or work evaluations) dropped because of drug or alcohol use? Have you ever been suspended or expelled (or fired) because of your drug or alcohol use? Have you often been high (or drunk) in situations when you knew you should have been straight?

2. Criterion. Recurrent substance use in physically hazardous situations.
   • **Clinical Questions**. Are you often high (or drunk) when it might be dangerous to you or someone else, such as when driving a car, operating a machine, or riding a bike?

3. Criterion. Recurrent substance-use–related legal problems.
   • **Clinical Questions.** Have you ever been in trouble with the law because of your drug or alcohol use? Do the police in your area know you as a drinker or drug user?

4. Criterion. Continued substance use despite persistent or recurrent social or interpersonal problems caused or exacerbated by the substance's effects.
   • **Clinical Questions.** Do people complain to you or worry about your substance use? Has your substance use gotten you in trouble with a boyfriend (or girlfriend, spouse, or friend)? Do people complain that your behavior gets out of control when you drink or use drugs?

DIAGNOSIS OF SUBSTANCE DEPENDENCE

The person must have experienced *three or more* of the following symptoms at any time *within a 12-month period*.

1. Criterion. Marked tolerance: The person usually needs at least 50% more of the substance to achieve intoxication or the desired effect, or the person experiences a markedly diminished effect with continued use of the same amount of the substance.
   • **Clinical Questions.** Have you found that it takes more of the substance to get high than it used to? When you first started using the substance, how much did it take to get high? How much does it take now?

2. Criterion. Withdrawal: The characteristic withdrawal syndrome for the particular substance has been experienced, or the same substance (or one from the same class or having cross addiction) is used to relieve or avoid the withdrawal symptoms.
   • **Clinical Questions (for alcohol).** Have you ever had the shakes or felt sick the morning after drinking, when you cut

down on the amount you drank, or when you stopped drinking altogether for a while? Have you ever experienced any of the following problems after stopping or cutting down on your drinking: sweating; racing heart; hand tremor; trouble sleeping; nausea; vomiting; seeing, feeling, or hearing things that others do not or that you know are not there; feeling agitated or wanting to pace; nervousness; or seizures? Have you ever used alcohol to get rid of the shakes or relieve a hangover?

Other drugs that produce withdrawal syndrome are amphetamines, cocaine, nicotine, opioids, sedatives, hypnotics, and anxiolytics (benzodiazepines, carbamates, barbiturates, barbiturate-like hypnotics). These drugs produce a variety of withdrawal symptoms. It is more manageable and simpler to ask the following.

- **Clinical Questions (for other drugs).** Have you ever felt physically sick when you cut down or stopped using the drug? Have you ever used the drug to relieve or avoid feeling sick?

TREATMENT

Many variables impact treatment outcomes. Although controversy exists over the most effective treatment methods, some clinicians agree that certain *patient variables* predict better results. The variables include:

- Absence of significant psychopathology (co-morbidity with other mental illness)
- Motivation (external motivation often prompts people to seek treatment, but internal motivation makes for lasting change)
- Social stability
- Stable marriage
- Stable job
- High socioeconomic status
- Positive social resources (people and organizations that support the person's sobriety)
- Low level of environmental stressors
- Varied and extensive repertoire of coping skills
- Length of time in treatment (continued involvement seems more important than the particular type of treatment)

The basic goals of treatment for substance abuse and substance dependence are different, yet compatible. For *substance abuse*, the intent of treatment is to *moderate use and reduce the risk and occurrence of problems*. This may be modified when there is every indication that the patient will progress to substance dependence (when illicit drugs are used) or when the patient is a child or adolescent. For *substance dependence*, the intent of treatment is to *achieve and maintain abstinence*. The patient should be able to *function comfortably* in his or her own environment without the use of drugs or alcohol. This is accomplished through various techniques that enhance motivation to initiate and maintain abstinence and by providing habilitation, for the patient who has never gained certain skills, or rehabilitation, for the patient who has lost skills as a result of their substance use, to assist in creating a life style that supports recovery.

The elements of treatment include:

- Employing techniques to maximize motivation
- Optimizing medical functioning (by treating withdrawal or other consequences of substance use)
- Identifying and treating other concurrent psychiatric symptoms or disorders
- Teaching skills for building a substance-free life style
- Teaching skills for enhancing and repairing relationships with family and friends
- Teaching skills for improving employment and management of money
- Addressing spiritual issues (by making connections to things larger than ourselves, such as the community or church)
- Teaching relapse awareness and prevention skills.

These elements of treatment may be delivered in several settings:

- Outpatient setting (usually 1 hour a week in individual or group therapy)
- Intensive outpatient setting (usually 3–4 hours a day for 4–5 days a week)
- Residential setting (full-time inpatient care)

The choice of setting depends on multiple variables. Indicators for more intense residential or intensive outpatient treatment include:

- Concurrent psychiatric disorders or medical problems (whether or not they relate to the substance use)
- Poor recovery environment
- Poor motivation
- Repeated past failures with treatment of lower intensity

Treatment of Withdrawal from Alcohol

The signs and symptoms of alcohol withdrawal usually appear within the first 24–48 hours after reducing or ceasing protracted, heavy alcohol use. Patients' experiences differ a great deal when they stop using alcohol, and history is one of the best predictors. Patients may experience none, some, or all of the following signs and symptoms. To meet the *DSM-IV* criteria, at least two of the signs and symptoms must be present, they must cause clinically significant impairment, and they must not be a result of or better accounted for by another medical condition. The signs and symptoms are:

- Autonomic hyperactivity (i.e., elevations in temperature and blood pressure)
- Hand tremor
- Insomnia
- Nausea, vomiting
- Psychomotor agitation
- Anxiety
- Visual, tactile, or auditory hallucinations or illusions
- Grand mal seizures

The severity of withdrawal occurs on a continuum, from minor discomfort to the more severe and life-threatening delirium tremens (DTs). DTs are characterized by:

- Clouding of consciousness
- Severe confusion
- Agitation
- Difficulty with attention
- Disorientation
- Perceptual problems
- Autonomic hyperactivity

Withdrawal from alcohol is treated on both an inpatient or outpatient basis. The level of medical management and nursing care needed is the deciding factor. Medical treatment typically consists of administering a drug that is cross-addictive to alcohol, usually a long-acting (i.e., chlordiazepoxide) or short-acting (ox-azepam, lorazepam) benzodiazepine. The condition of the liver determines which benzodiazepine to use. Impaired liver function makes a long-acting benzodiazepine more likely to accumulate and cause severe lethargy, drowsiness, and ataxia. When liver function is not a consideration, long-acting benzodiazepines often make the patient more comfortable and provide a smoother withdrawal. In addition to the medications used to treat withdrawal, thiamine, folic acid, and a multivitamin should be given to prevent the exacerbation of Wernicke-Korsakoff syndrome. The patient also must be put on bed rest and given proper nutrition.

EPIDEMIOLOGIC DATA

- Alcohol-related disorders are by far the most common substance-related disorders in the United States. More than 60% of adults between the ages of 21 and 45 are current alcohol users.
- Those aged 18–25 years are most likely to drink heavily, and a quarter of these individuals also take illicit drugs.
- The lifetime prevalence for alcohol abuse is approximately 20% of men and 10% of women.
- The lifetime prevalence for alcohol dependence is approximately 10% of men and 3%–5% of women.
- Approximately one-third of persons with alcohol dependence recovers without formal intervention, one-third improves with treatment, and one-third continues drinking until death.

CASE STUDY: MAN WITH ALCOHOL DEPENDENCE

A 41-year-old man was referred by his attorney for evaluation of his alcohol use. Apparently while intoxicated he struck his wife during an argument. She subsequently called the police, and he was arrested on domestic battery charges. He was annoyed that the court system was involved but was willing to comply with his attorney's request for the evaluation. He reported that he had his first drink at the age of 12 and was drinking regularly by the age of 15. He indicates that, at that time, he was drinking virtually every weekend, usually to intoxication. He stated that early on he could "hold his liquor" and rarely suffered hangovers. He reported that this pattern continued unchanged while in high school. After graduation he enlisted in the Army, and his drinking then increased significantly, both in volume and in frequency. He was reprimanded several times as a result of drinking-related incidents. He would often begin drinking in the morning and continue throughout the day when he had light duty. He found that he could not always predict when he would drink or how much. He was ordered by his commanding officer to participate in an alcohol treatment program but continued to drink. He was given a general discharge after 2 years of service. Following his discharge, he married, obtained employment, and has held the same job for nearly 20 years. He stated that there have been times when he has seriously tried to cut down or stop his drinking, mostly at the insistence of his wife, but has ultimately failed. He reported that he has had two DUI citations, the last one received 6 years ago. He indicated that in the morning he has a fine tremor that is relieved by alcohol. He denied regular use of illicit drugs but did report experimenting with cannabis while in the service. He reported a 20-year smoking habit of one to two packs of cigarettes a day.

After his attorney advised him that the charges of domestic battery would be dropped if he participated in an alcohol program, he was admitted to a general medical floor of the local hospital and treated for alcohol withdrawal. He was then transferred to a residential substance abuse facility, where he stayed for 14 days. His treatment consisted of enhancing his motivation, developing skills to maintain sobriety, repairing his family relationships, and introducing him to Alcoholics Anonymous (AA). Following the residential care, he participated in weekly outpatient therapy with a substance abuse counselor for 2 months, attended AA, and was able to remain sober.

MAJOR CLASSES OF COMMONLY ABUSED SUBSTANCES

The major classes of abused substances most commonly encountered are summarized below. The summary includes examples of specific substances within each class, typical routes of administration, intoxication and withdrawal states, detoxification guidelines, and epidemiologic data.

Amphetamine and Amphetamine-like Substances

Amphetamine and amphetamine-like substances increase neurotransmitter and electrical activity in the central nervous system (CNS). The dominant amphetamines used in the United States are methamphetamine (Desoxyn), methylphenidate (Ritalin), and dextroamphetamine (Dexedrine). Illicit users refer to them by a variety of street names, typically "speed," "crystal," "crystal meth," and "ice." When in doubt, ask the patient to name the drug if the street name is unfamiliar. The amphetamine-like drugs such as ephedrine and propranolamine, available in over-the-counter preparations, are less potent than the classic amphetamines. Other amphetamine-like drugs, referred to as "designer" amphetamines (MDMA is known as "ecstasy" or "Adam," MDEA is known as "Eve," DOM is called "STP"), exert combined stimulant and hallucinogenic effects.

ROUTES OF ADMINISTRATION

The routes of administration in order of quickness of action are: smoking, 7–10 seconds before effects are felt; injection, 15–30 seconds in the vein, 3–5 minutes in a muscle or under the skin; snorting, 3–5 minutes; and oral, 20–30 minutes.

INTOXICATION

At low-to-moderate doses, patients present with increased heart rate, increased respirations, elevated blood pressure, CNS stimulation, increased body temperature, appetite suppression, and euphoria. High doses may produce tachycardia or bradycardia, nausea, vomiting, muscular weakness, chest pain, and confusion.

WITHDRAWAL STATE

Users typically refer to the postintoxication state as a "crash." This consists of anxiety, tremulousness, dysphoric mood, lethargy, fatigue, nightmares, headache, profuse sweating, muscle cramps, stomach cramps, and cravings. These symptoms generally peak in 2–4 days and typically resolve within 1 week. The most dangerous symptom, particularly following a lengthy "run" or period of sustained amphetamine use, is depression accompanied by suicidal ideation and intent. These depressive feelings can last from weeks to months.

DETOXIFICATION GUIDELINES

In most cases supportive care is adequate, and medications are not required.

EPIDEMIOLOGIC DATA

More than 2% of the population has tried amphetamines, and those 18–25 years of age report the highest level of use. Smokable forms of amphetamines are currently popular in the United States, mostly on the East and West Coasts.

Cannabis

Cannabis is a hemp plant (*Cannabis sativa*) that contains many psychoactive cannabinoids; delta 9 tetrahydrocannabinol (THC) is the most potent.

ROUTES OF ADMINISTRATION

The cannabis plant is usually dried, chopped, and either rolled into cigarettes (joints) or smoked in a pipe. Cannabis also may be used in food or drinks, although the onset takes longer and the effects are less intense.

INTOXICATION

The effects of cannabis are dose dependent. At lower doses it produces a sedating effect with some mild confusion. Stronger doses produce giddiness; stimulation with increased alertness; increased appetite; and distortions of time, sound, and other sensations. Very strong doses can produce hallucinations. Physical symptoms include injected conjunctivae, dry mouth, and tachycardia.

WITHDRAWAL STATES

Although many users exhibit psychological dependence to cannabis, data are insufficient to support the existence of classic physical dependence. However, tolerance to many of the drug's effects has been demonstrated.

DETOXIFICATION GUIDELINES

If symptoms do appear, such as cravings for the drug, irritability, anxiety, or sleeplessness, expect them to be limited and responsive to supportive care.

EPIDEMIOLOGIC DATA

Cannabis is the most commonly used illicit drug. When smoked, the effects appear within minutes, peak in 30 minutes, and last from 2–4 hours. A variety of strengths (THC content) of cannabis are currently available, the strongest reaching 14% THC.

CASE STUDY: YOUNG MAN WITH CANNABIS ABUSE

The patient was a 17-year-old man brought to treatment by his parents after they found cannabis in the young man's room. He was initially angry that he had to come but became more open after realizing that the interview would be confidential and would not include his parents. He stated that he began using cannabis at the age of 12 and developed a regular use pattern by the age of 14. He smoked with his friends 1–2 times a week, mostly on the weekends. He got caught at school with cannabis 6 months ago and promised his parents he would never use cannabis again. He and his family agreed to participate in treatment, which consisted of individual and family therapy. After several weeks, he decided to abstain when he realized his parents would no longer allow him to drive the family car if he was going to use cannabis. Random toxicology testing along with firm parental guidelines has helped him remain drug free.

Cocaine

Cocaine is the most addictive of the major classes of abused substances. Cocaine powder is often referred to as "snow," "coke," "girl," or "lady." A freebase, smokeable form of cocaine is referred to as "crack" or "rock."

ROUTES OF ADMINISTRATION

Cocaine is used intranasally, by injection, or by smoking. When it is used intranasally (snorted), finely chopped cocaine powder is inhaled into the nose and absorbed through the nasal mucosa. When injected, the most common route of entry is the vein but is occasionally subcutaneous. Smoking is becoming the most common method of use because it delivers the drug to the brain within 10 seconds. It may also produce addiction more rapidly than any other route of administration.

INTOXICATION

Cocaine produces elation, euphoria, heightened self-esteem, and a sense of improved performance of mental and physical tasks. Higher doses can induce agitation, irritability, impaired judgment, hypersexuality, aggression, and increased psychomotor activity. The physical symptoms are tachycardia, pupillary dilation, hypertension, and mydriasis.

WITHDRAWAL STATES

The cessation of cocaine use is associated with dysphoria, anhedonia, anxiety, irritability, agitation, craving for the drug, and fatigue. For persons who use a relatively low-to-moderate amount, these symptoms typically abate within 24 hours. Persons who are heavy users or who have been using for long periods of time have symptoms that peak in 2–3 days but can persist for weeks.

DETOXIFICATION GUIDELINES

As with amphetamines, treatment typically consists of supportive care. Most clinicians avoid using medications unless absolutely necessary. Pharmacologic approaches to detoxification are being examined. Trials have been conducted with carbamazepine (Tegretol) and sympathomimetics such as methylphenidate (Ritalin).

EPIDEMIOLOGIC DATA

Cocaine use is highest among those between the ages of 18 and 25. It usually sells for $100–$150 a gram in most cities. On a per dose basis, that price is approximately 5–15 times higher than the cost of amphetamines.

CASE STUDY: A WOMAN WITH COCAINE DEPENDENCE

A 27-year-old woman was brought to the emergency room by the local police following a disturbance at her home. Apparently, she had secluded herself for several days and was threatening her neighbors. During questioning, she indicated that she thought people were trying to hurt her and she needed to protect herself. Her physical examination revealed significant weight loss within the last month, mucosal excoriations, needle marks, dilated pupils, and elevated blood pressure, heart rate, and temperature. She had no history of psychiatric problems, and her toxicology test revealed the presence of cocaine. She was admitted to the psychiatric floor of the hospital for observation. Her paranoid thoughts relented after 2 days, and she was transferred to the substance abuse unit. She participated in individual, group, and family counseling for her cocaine dependence. She was able to stay drug free and has had no recurrence of paranoid thought.

Hallucinogens

There are as many as 100 synthetic and naturally occurring hallucinogens. Examples of common, naturally occurring hallucinogens are psilocybin ("magic mushrooms") and mescaline ("peyote"). The most commonly used synthetic hallucinogen is lysergic acid diethylamide (LSD).

ROUTE OF ADMINISTRATION

Both synthetic and naturally occurring hallucinogens are most often used orally.

INTOXICATION

The response to this type of drug varies significantly, depending on the setting in which it is used and the personality of the user. The most common experiences are perceptual changes that occur while fully alert. These may consist of depersonalization, derealization, illusions, hallucinations, and synesthesias (seeing sound, hearing colors). Physical signs may include pupillary dilation, tachycardia, sweating, palpitations, and tremor.

WITHDRAWAL STATES

Tolerance for hallucinogens develops quickly from prolonged use and reverses quickly as well. Classic physical dependence and withdrawal symptoms do not occur with hallucinogens. Frequent users may experience psychologic dependence, but this is rare.

DETOXIFICATION GUIDELINES

There is no formal withdrawal state for persons on hallucinogens. Most management problems are related to intoxication or "bad trips," when patients experience significant anxiety, panic, and paranoia. Medications are rarely used. Patients should be placed in a nonthreatening, low-stimulus setting and offered reassurance. If necessary, a benzodiazepine can be administered, but an antipsychotic is rarely needed.

EPIDEMIOLOGIC DATA

Hallucinogens are classified as schedule I drugs with no medical use and high abuse potential. Those 18–25 years of age typically have the highest percentage of recent use. Hallucinogens are usually associated with less morbidity and mortality than other commonly used drugs. The popularity of these drugs is on the rise.

Inhalants

Inhalants are easily available, inexpensive, and in most cases legal. Solvents, glues, aerosol propellants, paint thinner, and fuels are commonly used.

Routes of Administration

As the name implies, this class of substances is inhaled through the nose or "huffed" through the mouth. Inhalants are rapidly absorbed through the lungs and delivered to the brain.

Intoxication

Depending on the specific substance used and the dose, the effects appear within 5 minutes and can last from 30 minutes to several hours. The inhalant user often appears to be drunk, showing signs of dizziness, nystagmus, incoordination, slurred speech, and unsteady gait. Behavioral and psychologic changes such as impulsiveness, belligerence, impaired judgment, and aggressiveness also may occur. The key to identifying recent inhalant use is to notice rashes around the nose and mouth, unusual breath odors, or remnants of the substance (such as paint thinner) on the user's body or clothing.

Withdrawal States

No formal withdrawal syndrome is associated with the use of inhalants. However, some heavy and prolonged users, upon cessation, complain of irritability, sleep disturbance, anxiety, nausea, tachycardia, and perceptual disturbances.

Detoxification Guidelines

Should the symptoms listed above occur, they are managed most often with supportive care alone.

Epidemiologic Data

Inhalant abuse is most often associated with youths aged 13–15 years. Currently, the largest group of users is in the eighth grade. Inhalant abuse is associated with many serious medical consequences including hepatic and renal damage. Death can result from respiratory depression, cardiac arrhythmias, asphyxiation, aspiration of vomitus, or an accident.

Nicotine

Nicotine is a psychoactive substance with euphoric and reinforcing qualities similar to cocaine and opioids. Tobacco is the most commonly used form of nicotine.

ROUTES OF ADMINISTRATION

Tobacco is smoked in cigarettes, cigars, and pipes. It can be chewed or used as snuff (finely chopped tobacco that is snorted or placed next to the gums so that the nicotine can be absorbed).

INTOXICATION

Nicotine has many effects but does not cause classic intoxication, defined as clinically significant maladaptive behavioral or psychologic changes as a result of the substance used. Users report reduced anxiety and improved attention, learning, reaction times, and mood.

WITHDRAWAL STATES

Withdrawal symptoms develop within 2 hours of the last use of nicotine and peak in 24–48 hours. Some protracted symptoms, if they occur, may last for weeks. Typical symptoms include intense cravings, irritability, increased frustration, anxiety, poor concentration, dysphoria, sleep disturbance, increased appetite and subsequent weight gain, muscle tension, and restlessness.

DETOXIFICATION GUIDELINES

Withdrawal and treatment of tobacco dependence is managed with a variety of nicotine replacement agents. These include the transdermal patch, nasal inhaler, or nicotine gum. Several other psychopharmacologic agents have been approved for the treatment of nicotine dependence or are effective in reducing withdrawal symptoms. These are clonidine, some antidepressants (fluoxetine, bupropion), and buspirone.

EPIDEMIOLOGIC DATA

Approximately 30% of the population over the age of 12 smoke tobacco. Although nicotine is a profoundly addictive drug, more than 90% of individuals who successfully stop using tobacco do so without formal intervention.

CASE STUDY: MAN WITH NICOTINE DEPENDENCE

The patient is a 64-year-old man who was referred by his cardiologist for treatment of his 50-plus-year tobacco habit. He stated that he smoked on average 1½–2 packs of cigarettes a day. He has made many failed attempts to stop smoking in the past at the insistence of his wife. When he was able to abstain, he experienced irritability, increased anxiety, restlessness, intense cravings, and headache. Treatment consisted of both psychologic and pharmacologic methods. His motivation was enhanced and maintained with counseling. He was encouraged to discuss the loss he felt giving up cigarettes, as well as his fears about his health. He used nicotine replacement therapy to address his physical addiction. After 3 months of abstinence, he found himself still thinking about smoking, but with supportive counseling he was able to remain nicotine free.

Opioids

The term opioid typically refers to the naturally occurring or semisynthetic and synthetic narcotic preparations that resemble an opiate in action. Examples of naturally occurring opioids are morphine, codeine, and thebaine. From these compounds, semisynthetics such as hydrocodone and acetaminophen (Vicodin), oxycodone and aspirin (Percodan), and heroin are produced. Synthetics include drugs such as meperidine (Demerol), propoxyphene (Darvon), and methodone (Dolophine).

Routes of Administration

The opioids may be taken orally, smoked, or injected intravenously or subcutaneously.

Intoxication

Physical signs of intoxication include pupillary constriction, drowsiness, slurred speech, and impaired memory or attention. Psychologic effects include euphoria and a sense of well-being.

Withdrawal States

Withdrawal from opioids can be painful but is rarely life-threatening. The general rule governing withdrawal from opioids is that short-acting drugs produce short but intense syndromes, while long-acting drugs produce prolonged and mild syndromes. Typically, mild-to-moderate withdrawal resembles the flu. Symptoms that may be seen include anxiety, dysphoria, yawning, sweating, rhinorrhea, lacrimation, piloerection, hypertension, and insomnia. With more severe withdrawal, symptoms may include deep muscle and joint pain, vomiting, diarrhea, and abdominal pain.

Detoxification Guidelines

Withdrawal is managed by two distinct methods, depending on the severity of the addiction and the expected symptoms. Patients experiencing less severe withdrawal are managed symptomatically with nonopiates such as clonidine and nonsteroidal anti-inflammatory drugs (NSAIDs). Subjectively, patients often complain that this method provides incomplete relief from discomfort. For patients experiencing more severe withdrawal, long-acting opiates are substituted for short-acting ones, then tapered over a period of days or weeks. Opiates tapered for a longer period typically provide a more comfortable withdrawal and better overall compliance. Currently, a variety of protocols are available to manage opioid withdrawal.

EPIDEMIOLOGIC DATA

The male-to-female ratio of opioid dependence is 3:1. Heroin is the most commonly abused opioid. It costs an individual hundreds of dollars a day to support a habit; thus, those addicted to heroin often turn to criminal activities. The rates of lifetime heroin use are highest among those aged 26–34 years. As the rate of human immunodeficiency virus (HIV) infection has increased as a result of contaminated needles, smoking has become a popular method of ingesting heroin. The smokable form is more potent than the injectable and results in people becoming addicted more rapidly.

CASE STUDY: MAN WITH OPIOID DEPENDENCE

The patient is a 29-year-old divorced man who reported a 2-year history of intravenous heroin use. He was employed in his father's business but often called in sick. His ex-wife has custody of their 3-year-old daughter.

He stated that he began using heroin at the prompting of a college friend, occasionally, at first, when he could afford the $30 to $50 it took to get high. Gradually, he found himself using more and more often, injecting 1–3 times a day. He complained of anxiety, sweating, lacrimation, rhinorrhea, and irritability when he could not obtain the drug. He admitted frequent visits to the emergency room attempting to obtain drugs. He indicated that before he started treatment he was using $100 worth of heroin a day. He was detoxified on a medical floor and transferred directly to an inpatient substance abuse program, but he left the program before completion and returned to heroin use. Following an arrest for drug possession 3 months later, he was ordered by the court to participate again in treatment. He successfully completed the program with the encouragement of the court and his family. He participates in outpatient counseling and attends Narcotics Anonymous. He has been drug free for 8 months.

Phencyclidine

Phencyclidine (PCP) is classified as a dissociative anesthetic. On the street, it is known as "angel dust," "crystal," "WAC," and "horse trangs."

ROUTES OF ADMINISTRATION

PCP can be ingested orally, taken intranasally, smoked (often mixed with cannabis), or injected.

INTOXICATION

Behavioral symptoms from PCP intoxication are aggressiveness, impulsiveness, and volatile emotions. Affect ranges from euphoria at low doses to extreme anxiety at high doses. Distorted perceptions and confusion are common. PCP intoxication is occasionally difficult to distinguish from the effects of hallucinogens. The major clue is numbness of the extremities resulting from the anesthetic qualities of the drug. Associated physical symptoms include muscle rigidity, ataxia, hypertension, tachycardia, and vertical or horizontal nystagmus.

WITHDRAWAL STATES

Tolerance to the effects of PCP has been demonstrated in humans, but most agree that physical dependence rarely develops.

DETOXIFICATION GUIDELINES

Since physical dependence rarely occurs, no accepted protocol exists for treatment. Most treatment of abstinence states consists of supportive and symptomatic care.

EPIDEMIOLOGIC DATA

PCP is often misrepresented on the street and sold as some other substance, usually THC, mescaline, or amphetamine. Most users are men between the ages of 20 and 40.

Sedatives, Hypnotics, and Anxiolytics

This group of substances contains a variety of drugs including benzodiazepines (diazepam [Valium], chlordiazepoxide [Librium], alprazolam [Xanax]), barbiturates (secobarbital [Seconal], pentobarbital [Nembutal]), and barbiturate-like drugs (Quaalude, glutethimide [Doriden], ethchlorvynol [Placidyl]). Sedatives are designed to bring about mental calmness, hypnotics induce sleep, and anxiolytics (similar to sedatives) decrease anxiety.

ROUTES OF ADMINISTRATION

These drugs are most commonly ingested orally. Some also may be used intravenously and intramuscularly.

INTOXICATION

This group of drugs produces a general depression of physiologic functions. The effects include sedation, slurred speech, nystagmus, diminished anxiety, euphoria, incoordination, disinhibition, mood lability, and depressed respiration.

WITHDRAWAL STATES

Withdrawal from benzodiazepines and barbiturates is similar to that from alcohol. The withdrawal symptomatology is typically a mixture of psychologic and physical problems. Patients develop tremor, gastrointestinal (GI) upset, muscle aches, increased pulse and respiration, elevated temperature, variable blood pressure, irritability, dysphoria, and anxiety. The severity of these symptoms depends on the half-life of the drug, the dose, and the duration of daily use. The onset of withdrawal from long-acting sedatives may be delayed for days following the last use, while short-acting drugs may produce withdrawal symptoms within hours of the last use. Withdrawal from these substances can be life-threatening.

DETOXIFICATION GUIDELINES

Detoxification from these drugs is complicated and should take place in an inpatient setting. Treatment involves giving the patient a cross-addictive drug with a longer half-life. The drug is administered over several days, then the dose is slowly tapered. A variety of protocols are available to manage withdrawal from specific drugs.

EPIDEMIOLOGIC DATA

Approximately 15% of the population in the United States have been or will be prescribed a benzodiazepine. Women are somewhat more likely to use and abuse these drugs. A prescription can inadvertently lead to drug abuse, as physicians tend to overprescribe benzodiazepines.

CHAPTER 11
Child and Adolescent Disorders

David H. Decker, M.D.

This chapter addresses two diagnostic classifications—mood disorders and disruptive behavior disorders. Examples are given of the diagnostic process for determining major depressive disorder (MDD) and attention-deficit/hyperactivity disorder (ADHD) as they are frequently encountered in children and adolescents and are often treated by primary care physicians.

MOOD DISORDERS

The diagnostic criteria for these disorders in children are the same as for adults, which have been described in an earlier chapter. The suggested referral strategies for mood disorders are discussed below.

- **Bipolar Disorder.** Children with bipolar disorders should be referred to a child and adolescent psychiatrist.
- **Dysthymia.** Children with dysthymia should be referred to a family therapist. The primary care physician should consider treating the patient pharmacologically, exactly as major depressive disorder is treated, and should consider referring the patient to a child and adolescent psychiatrist.
- **Adjustment Disorder.** Children and adolescents with adjustment disorder should not need medical treatment, but psychotherapy may be helpful.
- **Major Depressive Disorder (MDD).** The primary care physician may attempt to treat the patient initially pharmacologically. The physician should refer the child to a family therapist for behavioral problems and to a child and adolescent psychiatrist if the patient fails to respond after approximately 4 weeks on an adequate dose of antidepressant medication.

Major Depressive Disorder

CHIEF COMPLAINT

The chief complaint is usually presented by a parent:

- "He does not seem happy."
- "He is irritable."
- "Her schoolwork has deteriorated."

- "He has changed friends (or activities)."
- "She is withdrawn."
- "She does not go out like she used to."

DIFFERENTIAL DIAGNOSIS

The physician must exclude the following possibilities before diagnosing MDD in a child.

- Substance abuse can easily follow MDD as well as mimic it.
- Endocrine disorders are less likely to occur in children than in adults but are possible.
- Other disorders, such as seizure disorder, mononucleosis, and anemia should be excluded.
- Disruptive behavior disorders can coexist with or follow MDD.
- If the patient's symptoms meet diagnostic criteria for MDD, then the patient is not experiencing normal adolescence.

The physician must perform a complete medical and physical examination, including a complete blood count (CBC), Chem 20, urinalysis (UA), thyroid study, urine drug screen, electrocardiogram (ECG) [if considering tricyclic antidepressant use], and neurologic studies as indicated.

DIAGNOSIS

Five of the following nine symptoms must be present for more than 2 weeks in order to diagnose a major depressive episode. The patient or the parents can be asked the clinical questions. Since children and adolescents are notoriously poor at identifying their own feelings, obtaining the history from collateral sources is critical. The child should also be asked, but his or her answers should not be relied upon when they are negative.

1. **Criterion.** The patient is depressed or irritable most of the time nearly every day.
   - **Clinical Questions.** Is he or she withdrawn or sad, even on weekends or during the summer? Is he or she irritable, even with his or her friends? Is he or she angry most of the time?
   - **Clinical Observations.** The patient appears sad or simply unanimated during the interview.

2. **Criterion.** The patient has diminished interest or pleasure in most activities. Children and adolescents often compensate by increasing their pursuit of pleasure or changing to more intense (and often more dangerous) activities such as driving at high speeds, taking drugs, or listening to loud music.
   - **Clinical Questions.** Have hobbies or extracurricular activities

changed? (Often the child has another explanation such as, "I didn't like the coach." Unless most of the other students also quit the activity, this is insufficient to explain the change in most cases.) Are you able to have fun with your family or just doing simple things? Do you get bored easily, and is this a change? Tell me what you do for fun.

- **Clinical Observations.** The adolescent has no interest in conversation or interactions that might be amusing to a person of his age group.

3. Criterion. The patient has a change in appetite. This is rarely seen in children or adolescents, and it is difficult to determine if it is pathologic or a normal variation. Dramatic changes are most likely meaningful.

- **Clinical Questions.** How is your appetite? Has it changed recently?

4. Criterion. The patient has a change in sleep pattern. Parents are often unaware of their child's sleep pattern. The psychiatrist should ask specific questions. Children may simply refuse to stay in bed if they cannot fall asleep. A change in sleeping pattern is significant.

- **Clinical Questions.** What time do you go to bed? What time do you go to sleep? Do you wake up during the night? What time do you get up?

5. Criterion. The patient has psychomotor agitation or retardation. This is rarely seen in children who occasionally become more active as they become more tired.

- **Clinical Questions.** Has the child's activity level changed? Does he or she show the same energy he or she used to?
- **Clinical Observations.** The child responds slowly to fairly simple questions and is irritable.

6. Criterion. The child exhibits fatigue.

- **Clinical Questions.** What is the child's activity level, and has it changed? What does his or her typical day include?
- **Clinical Observations.** The child appears tired or bored.

7. Criterion. The child has feelings of worthlessness and guilt. These feelings are difficult for an adolescent to identify.

- **Clinical Questions.** Do you feel worthless? Do you feel guilt about anything? (Guilt is often out of proportion to the event.)
- **Clinical Observations.** The child has poor eye contact and tends not to defend him- or herself appropriately when challenged.

8. Criterion. The child has a diminished ability to concentrate.

- **Clinical Questions.** How is your concentration? Is it harder to do your schoolwork than it used to be? Have your grades changed? Do you find yourself daydreaming more?
- **Clinical Observations.** The child loses his or her place when asked to count serial 7s. He or she may lose track of lengthy questions.

9. Criterion. The child has thoughts of suicide or death. Children and adolescents *do* have these thoughts and *do* successfully commit suicide!

- **Clinical Questions.** Have you ever thought of hurting yourself? Have you ever thought of killing yourself? Have you ever wished you were dead or were never born? Do you feel everyone would be better off without you? If the child answers "yes" to any of these questions, he or she should be referred to a psychiatrist.

SUMMARY

Questions must be asked in multiple ways to obtain important information that the patient or family may be reluctant to give. The physician may have concerns about biasing the responses with this technique. To prevent bias, review the positive responses in detail with the patient and family to delete those answers given to please the interviewer.

Parents and clinicians tend to "normalize" the behaviors described. Deviant behavior or psychiatric illness can be overlooked or excused by statements such as "Oh, he's just being a teenager."

Adolescence does not have to be traumatic. Healthy teenagers do not manifest significant dysfunction at school or home. Mood changes related to boyfriends or girlfriends or other social factors do not meet the criteria for MDD.

CASE STUDY: ADOLESCENT WITH MDD

A 14-year-old boy was brought in by his parents for an evaluation. The parents complained that their son's grades were worsening and he was becoming increasingly disrespectful to them. The patient denied feeling sad but admitted he was somewhat irritable at home, at school, and with his friends, although mostly with his parents. His grades had fallen from As and Bs to Cs and Ds. He described an initial sleep delay of 1 hour for the past 3 months. He did not try out for basketball this year, even though his parents stated that he was one of the best players in his class last year. He continues to go out with his friends, but his parents feel he initiates fewer contacts now than he did previously. He admits to being easily bored, and his parents believe that his motivation and energy level seem fairly low, stating, "He's gotten pretty lazy this year."

Treatment
Pharmacologic Therapy

Early studies did not support the pharmacologic treatment of depressive disorders in children and adolescents; however, recent studies of newer antidepressants have been encouraging. Most child psychiatrists agree that a trial of antidepressants benefits children with MDD. A good rule for pediatric pharmacology is to try to use medications that have at least a 5-year history of use in adults without significant adverse effects.

Tricyclic antidepressants have been available for many years and are effective; however, physicians have expressed concerns about cardiac arrhythmias and the high lethality from overdoses seen in the younger population. These medications are thus a second choice following use of newer serotonin-reuptake inhibitors (SSRIs) such as fluoxetine, sertraline, and paroxetine. Even newer formulations like venlafaxine, nefazodone, and mirtazapine should be considered prior to using the tricyclic antidepressants. Buproprion has also been studied fairly well in children, although its effect on lowering the seizure threshold is of concern. Monoamine oxidase inhibitors (MAOIs) should be prescribed only by a psychiatrist and for specific reasons with close monitoring.

Side effects of SSRIs are minimal but may include irritability, sedation, gastrointestinal (GI) upset, and vivid dreams or restless sleep. The chance of taking a lethal overdose is low. Consider administering lower doses of SSRIs than recommended, even for older adolescents, because of concerns that minor, annoying side effects may lead to more noncompliance than in the adult population. Dosage schedules are not available for children; however, children under 12 years of age should be given the lowest possible initial dose. The dose can be increased fairly rapidly, but the final level should be less than the usual effective dose for adults. Side effects should be monitored closely. Research on dosage schedules in children is currently being conducted.

Electroconvulsive therapy (ECT) is rarely considered as a result of poor scientific data on efficacy and side effects in developing children and the negative stigma attached to this form of treatment.

Psychotherapy

Psychotherapy should be part of treatment for nearly all cases of MDD. Mild cases may benefit from several weeks of therapy before a trial of medication is indicated. Patients who clearly have MDD with many obvious symptoms should be given medication for several weeks before psychotherapy is initiated, since it is time-consuming and expensive.

DISRUPTIVE BEHAVIOR DISORDERS

The suggested referral strategies are as follows.

- **Oppositional Defiant Disorder (ODD).** ODD is present when the patient exhibits a pattern of negativistic, hostile, and defiant behavior. Medication is not indicated for this condition. Referral to a family therapist is needed for the parents to learn important behavioral techniques. The individual should be referred to a child psychiatrist if treatment does not seem to help within a few weeks or months. ODD often is associated with other disorders such as MDD or ADHD.
- **Conduct Disorder.** Conduct disorder is present when the patient exhibits a persistent pattern of violating the basic rights of others and not adhering to the rules and norms of society. The causes and associated problems seen with conduct disorder are complex and varied. Family therapy may be appropriate for mild cases, but referral to a child psychiatrist should not be delayed in more difficult cases.
- **Attention-Deficit/Hyperactivity Disorder.** ADHD is often initially treated pharmacologically. Referral is appropriate to a psychotherapist or family therapist for behavioral interventions and the resolution of issues of self-esteem, frustration, and other secondary emotional factors. The child should be referred to a child psychiatrist if the initial response is poor or if other issues are complicating the case.

Attention-Deficit/Hyperactivity Disorder

CHIEF COMPLAINT

- "She is not doing well in school."
- "He does not behave."
- "He cannot stay in his seat."
- "He gets mad easily."
- "He is impulsive."
- "He is easily distracted."
- "He is lazy" (or "he could do it if he wanted to but he does not").
- "He is disorganized (or forgetful)."

DIFFERENTIAL DIAGNOSIS

The physician must exclude the following possibilities before diagnosing the child with ADHD.

- Lead toxicity
- Seizure disorder. Look for staring spells in the history.
- Depressive disorder or bipolar disorder. Depression may follow ADHD.
- Substance abuse. A history of ADHD as a child helps sort out these issues.
- Abuse, ongoing trauma, severe stress, or anxiety. Determine on what the child focuses instead of school work.
- Conduct disorder or ODD. Often, both ADHD and either conduct disorder or ODD are present.
- Normal. Significant impairment in more than one setting excludes a diagnosis of normal.

DIAGNOSIS

Several criteria must be met for a diagnosis of ADHD:

- Symptoms must have been present prior to 7 years of age.
- Symptoms must be seen in at least two settings (e.g. at home or school).
- Six symptoms must be present among criteria 1–9 or criteria 10–18.
- Normal abilities for the child's age must be factored when determining the significance of impairment. All symptoms must occur often.

1. Criterion. The child fails to pay close attention to details and makes careless mistakes.
- **Clinical Questions.** Does he or she have difficulty following directions (without outright refusal), especially multistep directions? Does he or she seem to rush his or her work or make careless mistakes?
- **Clinical Observations.** The child makes random mistakes when given relatively easy calculations. The child does not pause when appropriate to think about the questions asked.

2. Criterion. The child has difficulty sustaining attention during tasks or play. At times, children learn to avoid activities that require sustained attention.
- **Clinical Questions.** Does your child get bored easily? Does he or she tend to switch activities often, even before the previous activity is completed?
- **Clinical Observations.** In a play setting, the child changes activities often, typically without completing the previous activity (e.g., he or she only completes half a puzzle). The child may complain that a play event is boring and stop to move on to another activity.

3. Criterion. The child does not seem to listen when spoken to directly. Do not include times when the child is engaged in video games or watching television.
- **Clinical Questions.** Does your child have difficulty listening? Does your child become over-focused and not seem to hear you when you address him or her?
- **Clinical Observations.** The child does not sustain focus when given instructions. Immediately following clearly articulated instructions or statements, the child may ask you to repeat them.

4. Criterion. Often he or she does not follow through on instructions or fails to finish tasks, duties, or homework (not because of opposition). This problem may occur even when it is clearly in the child's best interest to complete the tasks, such as when a promised reward follows.
- **Clinical Questions.** Does your child have more difficulty with multistep directions than other children his or her age? Does your child seem to get lost in the instructions if more than one is given? Does your child try to follow some instructions and get lost or distracted while doing so?
- **Clinical Observations.** The child gets confused by multistep directions. He or she fails to complete an assigned task in a reasonable amount of time.

5. Criterion. The child has difficulty organizing tasks or activities.
- **Clinical Questions.** Does your child seem disorganized?
- **Clinical Observations.** The child's desk, bookbag, and room are messy. He or she takes many things out without putting much away, leaving a cluttered play area.

6. Criterion. The child or adolescent avoids, dislikes, or is reluctant to engage in tasks that require sustained mental effort such as homework and schoolwork. This is often mistaken for opposition.
- **Clinical Questions.** Does your child have difficulty doing homework tasks, even when they are not too difficult? Does your child avoid playing games that require patience or waiting?
- **Clinical Observations.** Parental observation is necessary. The child avoids tasks to such a degree that he or she is willing to spend more time avoiding the work than the task would have originally required.

7. Criterion. The child loses objects that are necessary for tasks or activities.
- **Clinical Questions.** Does your child tend to lose or misplace

things? Does your child do homework but sometimes fail to turn it in?

- **Clinical Observations.** Parental observation is necessary. The child may misplace things in plain sight and may "lose" common items such as his or her shoes.

8. Criterion. The child or adolescent is easily distracted. This generally refers to external distraction. The physician should look for a depressive disorder if the child seems internally distracted.

- **Clinical Questions.** Is your child more easily distracted than other children of this age? If your child is doing an activity (not a video), is he or she more aware of or distracted by the little noises around him or her than other children seem to be?
- **Clinical Observations.** The child shows distractibility during an interview by looking around whenever another noise is made, for instance, looking at the door if there is a noise outside the room.

9. Criterion. The child often forgets daily activities. Memory most likely is not the problem; he or she may be able to remember some things very well. The child simply cannot recall something to which he or she did not pay attention initially.

- **Clinical Questions.** Is your child more forgetful than other children? Does your child need frequent reminders?
- **Clinical Observations.** Typically this information can be obtained only from the history, unless a great deal of time is spent with the child.

10. Criterion. The child leaves his or her seat when he or she is expected to remain seated. This symptom occurs more often when demands for remaining seated become greater.

- **Clinical Questions.** Does your child have difficulty remaining seated? Can your child sit through an entire dinner without getting up?
- **Clinical Observations.** The child does not remain in his or her seat during the interview process, even if asked.

11. Criterion. He or she runs about or climbs excessively (the child feels restless).

- **Clinical Questions.** Does your child climb or run more than others his or her age? Does your child place him- or herself in danger by running, jumping, or climbing without reasonable care? Is your child accident prone? Does he or she often feel restless?
- **Clinical Observations.** The child may even climb about the chair during an interview and run into and out of the room.

12. Criterion. The child has difficulty playing quietly. These sounds are not always annoying to those around him or her and may include more "quiet" singing or humming.
- **Clinical Questions.** Does your child tend to be noisy or have difficulty playing without making noises?
- **Clinical Observations.** The child hums to him- or herself even while others are conversing. He or she makes many thumping or rapping noises while seated to amuse him- or herself.

13. Criterion. The child is always "on the go" or "driven by a motor."
- **Clinical Questions.** Does your child always tend to be doing something? Is your child able to just sit quietly and enjoy him- or herself? Is your child always on the go?
- **Clinical Observations.** The child is in continuous motion; as soon as one activity is stopped, another is begun.

14. Criterion. The adolescent or child fidgets or squirms. These children often "touch things too much."
- **Clinical Questions.** Is your child fidgety? Does your child always tend to have his or her hands or feet in motion, even when sitting in one place?
- **Clinical Observations.** The child's hands or feet are almost always in constant motion. They are always touching something or playing with their clothes or other accessible objects.

15. Criterion. He or she talks excessively.
- **Clinical Questions.** Is your child very verbal? Does your child talk too much at school?
- **Clinical Observations.** He or she is hyperverbal and really wants to talk, even though there is no important point to be made.

16. Criterion. The child blurts out answers.
- **Clinical Questions.** Does your child get in trouble for not raising his hand in class? Does your child blurt out answers without thinking about the question or before the question has been completed?
- **Clinical Observations.** He or she blurts out the answer or cannot wait until a question is completed before responding.

17. Criterion. The child has difficulty awaiting his or her turn. Children often get into the most trouble when waiting is required, such as poking their peers when standing in line.
- **Clinical Questions.** Does your child have difficulty waiting his or her turn or avoid playing games that require waiting for one's turn?

- **Clinical Observations.** The child tries to rush the therapist when it is his or her turn in a game, or he or she avoids games that require waiting.

18. **Criterion.** The child interrupts or intrudes.
    - **Clinical Questions.** Does your child tend to interrupt more than other children his or her age? Does your child tend not to wait for others to conclude conversations or interactions before he or she intrudes?
    - **Clinical Observations.** The child seems undersocialized; he or she has no qualms about intruding on interactions of others and interrupts often.

Summary

Parents often have adapted to their child's behavior and thus underestimate the difficulties these behaviors cause in other settings. Specific questioning is necessary in these situations. Avoid simply asking the parent if the child does too much of a certain behavior. Parents often have an agenda when their child is being evaluated for ADHD. For example, when asked how high their child's energy level is, they might respond, "He's not hyper." A frank discussion of ADHD and the implications of the evaluation may be needed. Parents and clinicians often grossly underestimate the psychologic sequelae of ADHD and find themselves thinking, "He could do it (behave and get good grades) if he wanted to." Unfortunately, the child is not doing "it." He or she is actually losing out on developing positive self-esteem and critical social skills while others are waiting for him or her to give more of an effort.

Case Study: Boy with ADHD

A 7-year-old boy was brought in for an evaluation by his parents after his teacher voiced some concerns to them. The teacher noted their son was doing somewhat poorly. He seemed easily distracted, had difficulty following directions, tended to have difficulty waiting his turn, and needed frequent reminders to raise his hand before responding. The parents noted that from a young age their son had always had a high-energy level, with his father stating proudly, "He's all boy." They admitted he was difficult at home. He had trouble following directions, refusing at times but also seeming to get lost in the instructions or while completing the task. He was verbally and physically impulsive. The parents were uncertain if this was just normal for his age, though it was moderately distressing to them.

TREATMENT

ADHD has many associated medical and psychologic problems. Unless the medication has a positive effect, the child should be referred to a mental health care provider for further assessment or services. The following suggestions focus on children with uncomplicated ADHD. Multimodal treatment is warranted for most patients. A comprehensive plan may include specialized school programming, behavioral interventions at home and school for conduct and organizational issues, specific training programs such as pro-social skills training, psychotherapy for the child and parents, and medication. Complex cases most likely require the services of multiple providers.

Stimulants

Stimulant medications such as methylphenidate (Ritalin) or dextroamphetamine (Dexedrine) are typically used because of their superior efficacy and side-effect profiles.

- *Methylphenidate* typically is chosen first because it has a slightly better side-effect profile. Methylphenidate has a short half-life, and for all-day coverage (recommended in most cases) at least three doses a day are needed, spaced approximately 3½–5 hours apart. The dosage varies, with a maximum of approximately 0.6 mg/kg/dose or 20 mg/dose (whichever is less). A reasonable rationale for exceeding this dose is a partial response with no significant side effects.
- *D-Amphetamine* dosage is usually approximately half that of methylphenidate and may last longer than the typical 4 hours for methylphenidate. Many side effects are managed by scheduling changes in the medication.

Antidepressants

Antidepressants including imipramine, desipramine (tricyclics), and buproprion effectively treat ADHD. Tricyclics must be closely monitored for possible cardiac side effects. The dosage is usually similar or less than that used in treating depression.

- *Clonidine* and *guanfacine* are commonly used as adjuncts when the initial response is positive, but impulsivity and hyperactivity remain problems. As concerns have been raised about possible cardiac effects from these medications when used with stimulants, physicians now recommend ECG monitoring.

CHAPTER 12
Delirium and Dementia

Terry A. Travis, M.D., M.S.Ed.

INTRODUCTION
Definition

Delirium and dementia are syndromes that reflect significant cognitive impairment. Cognition is one of the higher order processes of the brain. **It is imperative to recognize these syndromes, as the cause is often treatable.**

Chief Complaint

- "I get lost and cannot remember people and things I should."
- "My husband does not recognize friends and gets lost in the house."
- "My wife cannot keep track of what she is doing."
- "I cannot let my husband drive or handle the money anymore; he just cannot handle it."
- "My husband has become disoriented and fearful during the past day."
- "Since starting that medicine, my brother does not know where he is, is seeing things, and is afraid of people."
- "My mom almost sold the farm for 10% of its value."
- "Every evening, my wife starts calling me by another name, hitting me, and screaming about me hurting her."

Differential Diagnosis

To diagnose delirium or dementia, the cause must be determined. The following should be considered and excluded. Other psychiatric illnesses such as depression, schizophrenia, dissociative disorder, and factitious disorder usually can be excluded easily by taking a thorough history; the pattern of symptoms quickly rules out these disorders. Normal aging must be excluded as well. All medical conditions must be excluded, as any that affect brain function can cause these syndromes. Examples are:

- Infection (including HIV)
- Fever
- Metabolic disturbances such as those caused by renal or hepatic disease, hyper- or hypothyroidism, electrolyte imbalance, and hypoglycemia

- Head trauma such as concussion or subdural or epidural hematoma
- Intracranial lesions caused by cerebrovascular accident, cyst, neoplasm, or aneurysm
- Seizures
- Thiamine or vitamin B_{12} deficiency
- Cardiovascular problems such as hypotension, cardiac failure, or arrhythymia
- Intoxication or withdrawal from medication, poison, or substance of abuse
- Anemia
- Degenerative diseases such as Parkinson's, Huntington's, Pick's, and Creutzfeldt-Jakob diseases

To rule out potentially reversible causes, in addition to a thorough history and physical examination the following laboratory studies, often termed a delirium or dementia workup, should be done.

- Electroencephalogram (EEG)—generalized background slowing helps rule in the diagnosis of delirium
- Complete blood count (CBC)
- Blood urea nitrogen (BUN) and creatinine
- Liver function tests
- Blood glucose
- Erythrocyte sedimentation rate
- Electrolytes with calcium and magnesium
- Thyroid function tests
- Serology for syphilis
- Toxicology screen
- Chest x-ray
- Urinalysis
- Computed tomography (CT) or magnetic resonance imaging (MRI) of head
- Lumbar puncture, if indicated
- Human immunodeficiency virus (HIV) serology
- Heavy metal screening and bromide levels
- Serum vitamin B_{12}, folate, and thiamine levels

DELIRIUM

Diagnosis

Criteria for the diagnosis of delirium are discussed below.

1. Criterion. The patient exhibits a reduced and fluctuating level of consciousness and has problems maintaining contact with and attending to stimuli in the environment.

- **Clinical Questions.** Use the sensorium and mental capacity portion of the Mental Status Examination to document the patient's symptoms, including changes over time. The Mini-Mental Status Examination (MMSE) can be used to quantify the patient's level of function (see Chapter 2).

- **Clinical Observations.** While being interviewed, the patient stops responding or responds inappropriately to questions, then after a variable period of time, responds normally again. The patient may start picking at the bedding or bedclothes for no reason and may not react to the psychiatrist's presence or to whatever is occurring in the room. The patient may quickly and randomly switch from looking at and attending to the surroundings, to looking out the window, to looking at the television, to examining the pillow, or to picking something up off the nightstand.

2. **Criterion.** The patient has problems with cognition and perception, exhibiting disorientation, language disturbances, and hallucinations.
- **Clinical Questions.** Refer to clinical questions above for reduced levels of consciousness.
- **Clinical Observations.** The patient, when asked, says he or she is somewhere else and with other people. The patient may start using neologisms or words that do not make sense. The patient may describe hallucinations as if the psychiatrist can also observe them. At times the patient may become terrified and try to escape, run, or leave because of them.

3. **Criterion.** Delirium develops rapidly over a few hours to days, with a fluctuating course throughout the day.
- **Clinical Questions.** Refer to the clinical questions above for reduced levels of consciousness.
- **Clinical Observations.** All of these symptoms can vary over time, even from minute to minute, from severe to absent.

CASE STUDY: WOMAN WITH DELIRIUM

The patient was a 73-year-old married woman who was seen 3 days after a triple coronary artery bypass procedure. She had done well until the evening before when she became disoriented and agitated; she called the nurse two to three times and then forgot the reason for the call. Her blood gases were normal, and no abnormal laboratory findings were noted. She was on a variety of medications, several of which may have interacted and caused sedation. When interviewed by a medical student, her mental status was normal, and she gave a coherent, logical history and was cooperative and alert. Thirty minutes later she could not give appropriate answers to questions but talked over and over about the three men in her room who had crawled in through the window. She wondered how they did this as she was on the fifth floor (this was accurate) and said they talked about her, did not frighten her, and then left. She was unable to tell how they left. She said she was in the town she lived in 20 years ago and thought one of the physicians present was a surgeon who had operated on her. (She remembered something was done to her chest.) Her mental status varied from normal to abnormal, fluctuating from every 30 minutes to several hours. Her medications were reviewed and decreased to minimize sedation and interaction, and she was perfectly clear and her usual self within 24 hours.

Treatment

- The physician must find and treat the cause immediately. This is an emergency; delay can result in permanent cognitive impairment and possibly death in cases of withdrawal or reaction to drugs or toxins.
- Fluid and electrolyte balance and appropriate nutrition must be maintained.
- The patient should be observed closely for changes in vital signs.
- The physician should provide orienting stimuli in the room such as a family member or friend, a radio, a calendar, and reasonable lighting. Staff can re-orient the patient whenever they are in the room. This is particularly important to minimize the chance of "sundowning," the noticeable increase in delirium that often occurs in the evening. The patient's delirium may increase, with a concomitant increase in agitation or fear, as the visual stimulation decreases with lessening sunlight.
- The patient must not be overstimulated; this problem can occur in intensive care units.
- If the delirium is caused by withdrawal from alcohol or drugs, benzodiazepines should be administered.
- If agitation, psychosis, or fearfulness occur, low doses of haloperidol or risperidone should be given.

DEMENTIA

Diagnosis

There are two criteria for the diagnosis of dementia.

1. **Criterion.** Memory impairment is the major feature.
   - **Clinical Questions.** Refer to the clinical questions for reduced levels of consciousness.

- **Clinical Observations.** The patient does not remember the psychiatrist's name after a few minutes. The patient cannot remember or learn new information such as where he or she is and why. He or she gradually loses previously learned information. The loss of recent memories and learning is more severe than remote memory. The patient may not know where he or she is and get lost easily or may be unable to say where he or she is currently living, but he or she can discuss his or her time in the military and previous jobs and friends accurately. Remote memory gradually erodes until the patient no longer remembers names of family members or his or her own name.

2. Criterion. One of the following cognitive disturbances significantly impairs function. **Aphasia** is the misuse of words or the loss of ability to remember and use words correctly. **Apraxia** is the inability to perform motor activities even though the motor activity is intact. **Agnosia** is the inability to recognize objects even though the senses (sight, hearing, touch, taste, smell) are intact. **Loss of executive functioning** is the inability to think in the abstract, plan ahead to complete a task, or organize activities in sequence.

- **Clinical Questions.** Refer to the clinical questions for reduced levels of consciousness.
- **Clinical Observations.** Patients have a decreased ability to perform the activities of daily living (ADLs) such as bathing, cooking, shopping, and dressing. They have lost the ability to read, comprehend, and write. Patients may become lost and be unable to remember where they were going or how to get there. These patients also lose normal social inhibitions. The term "dirty old man" comes from the inappropriate sexual behaviors of demented patients. Patients exhibit a labile affect with sudden, inexplicable laughter or crying, as well as perseveration of speech.

Subtypes of Dementia

Dementia of the Alzheimer's type is characterized by a gradual onset and continuing cognitive decline, causing significant impairment. Vascular dementia is characterized by focal neurologic signs or laboratory evidence of multiple infarcts of the cortex and underlying white matter that appear to be etiologically related to the loss of function.

CASE STUDY: MAN WITH DEMENTIA

The patient is a 52-year-old man who was admitted to the psychiatry unit because of a change in his behavior. Over the past few months, he exhibited marked aggression and anger and would strike out at other residents of the nursing home where he lived. He was in the nursing home because of a disability associated with 40 years of severe insulin-dependent diabetes. He was noted to be disoriented, was unable to remember anything for more than 5 seconds, and was unable to do simple math. His Folstein MMSE score was 14/30. Routine laboratory studies showed that the patient's calcium level was high, and he was diagnosed with hyperparathyroidism. Within 12 hours after parathyroid gland surgery, he spontaneously remembered the physician's name after being reintroduced on rounds. His MMSE score was 28, and he returned to the nursing home "the same person we had always known."

CASE STUDY: MAN WITH DEMENTIA OF THE ALZHEIMER'S TYPE

The patient is a 74-year-old retired engineer who began having trouble remembering words and could not express himself clearly. He began to have increasing memory problems. A full evaluation revealed a MMSE score of 24 that had previously been 30. The patient was unable to find his way home at times when he rode his bicycle in his neighborhood, something he had done for many years. He was aware of when he became lost and was appropriately concerned. He continued to be socially pleasant but became more and more forgetful so that he could no longer cook for himself or plan what to wear, although he could still dress himself. He was told he had dementia resembling the Alzheimer's type, and he and his family made long-term plans for his care. His son visits several times a week, and a live-in caretaker currently resides with him. He is otherwise healthy.

Treatment

Since 15% of dementias are caused by a treatable condition, the first step involves fully evaluating the patient to discover the cause, and then providing appropriate treatment. Treatable dementia may result from:

- Head trauma
- Chronic subdural hematoma
- Normal-pressure hydrocephalus
- Intracranial tumors
- Vitamin deficiencies
- Endocrinopathies such as thyroid, parathyroid, adrenal, and pituitary disease
- Infections such as AIDS, syphilis, cerebral abscess, and chronic meningitis
- Heavy metal poisoning

- Drug toxicity from prescribed medications or alcohol and abused substances
- Metabolic problems such as dehydration, electrolyte disturbances, porphyria, renal or hepatic failure, Wilson's disease, or hypoxemia from any cause
- Collagen-vascular disease such as systemic lupus erythematosus, temporal arteritis, or sarcoidosis

The physician should symptomatically treat depression, psychosis, or insomnia. The patient and family should be taught about the changes that are occurring and the resources available through support groups. Appropriate environmental stimuli should be provided with things like television and newspapers. Daily schedules should be consistent, avoiding overstimulation and change. Other measures, listed under the treatment for delirium, are used for these types of dementias as well.

CHAPTER 13
Psychiatric Emergencies

Terry A. Travis, M.D., M.S.Ed.

SUICIDE

Of patients who commit or attempt suicide, 95% suffer from a common, readily diagnosable psychiatric disorder:

- Depressive disorder—50%
- Substance abuse—30%
- Schizophrenia—10%
- Delirium/dementia—5%

Two-thirds have told someone else about their suicidal thoughts, and one-half have seen a physician less than 1 month prior to their suicide.

Risk Factors

- Gender. Men are three times more successful in committing suicide, but women attempt suicide four times as often.
- Age. Men are generally older than 45 years of age, and women are generally older than 55 years. Over 65 years of age, men and women commit suicide at an equal rate.
- Race. Caucasians commit suicide at twice the rate of non-Caucasians.
- Marital status. Those who are alone because of divorce, being widowed, or never having married are at greater risk.
- Prior suicidal behavior is an important risk factor.
- Mental illness
- Loss of physical health (chronic illness in particular)
- Unemployed or retired
- Prior inpatient psychiatric care
- Significant anger, rage, or violence
- Recent significant stressor resulting in markedly changed circumstances

Assessment

All of the above risk factors should be assessed. If the patient expresses suicidal ideation, the physician should determine:

- If the thoughts are specific, vague, or just passing (the pervasiveness of the thoughts).

- If the thoughts are specific, what are the plans and how extensively have they been formulated? Has the patient done anything to carry them out such as buying a gun or accumulating drugs?
- The lethality of the plan and the availability of means to accomplish the plan.
- The probability of rescue if the proposed means are followed

AGITATION, AGGRESSION, AND VIOLENCE

Agitation, aggression, and violence have many causes, including:

- Acute drug or alcohol withdrawal
- Acute drug or alcohol intoxication
- Acute mania
- Delirium or dementia
- Acute psychoses
- Personality disorder (especially sociopathic)
- Acute post-traumatic stress disorder

Management

- Decrease the patient's stimulation by placing him or her in a quiet room or situation.
- Attempt to lessen the patient's agitation with a calm, soothing, and collaborative approach.
- Show available force by calling for security guards and other personnel.
- Help the patient verbalize his or her feelings.
- Tell the patient that every precaution will be taken so that he or she and others do not get hurt.
- Monitor your feelings. A physician who feels threatened should tell the patient this and the solution being proposed.
- The physician should always summon help; do *not* attempt to control the patient alone.
- A clear personal space should be maintained between the physician and patient.
- Do not block the door, as the patient should have the option of leaving.
- Medication can be offered as a means for the patient to gain control of his or her behavior.
- If violence is still threatened and appears imminent, apply physical or mechanical restraints as needed.
- Use medication without the patient's consent only when there is an immediate risk of injury to the patient or others.

CHAPTER 14
Forensic Psychiatry

Terry A. Travis, M.D., M.S.Ed.

CIVIL COMMITMENT

The patient must meet both of the following standards:

- The patient must have a mental illness.
- The patient must pose a risk of harm to self or to others:

  - By intentional harmful acts towards self (suicide or self-mutilation)
  - By the inability to safely meet the ordinary demands of daily life (not eating, not treating illnesses or infections, possibly freezing)
  - By intentional harmful acts towards others (homicidal or aggressive)

A physician or other health care provider (as defined by law) must complete the first legal documents for involuntary commitment. Typically, a psychiatrist must examine the patient, complete a second legal document for involuntary commitment, and then testify before a judge within 5 working days.

A formal hearing is held before a judge. The patient, family, interested others, attorneys, and the psychiatrist are present to give testimony. The judge must make a decision balancing the interests of society against the patient's interest in freedom.

COMPETENCY

To be declared competent, a person must meet all of the following legal standards:

- The person must be able to communicate a choice or decision.
- The person must understand the information that is needed to make the decision.
- The person must be able to manipulate the information rationally to make the decision.
- The person must be able to personally appreciate the situation involved in the decision and the potential consequences of the decision on that situation.

Once a person has been declared legally incompetent, either a guardian or conservator is appointed.

- A guardian is appointed to make decisions regarding the basic necessities of life.
- A conservator is appointed to make decisions regarding basic financial affairs.

Persons who are determined to be legally incompetent cannot sign contracts, including marriage and divorce contracts; make a will (testamentary capacity); drive a vehicle; handle their own property; or practice their profession. The psychiatric basis for providing evidence of incompetency is based on the person's inability to make proper judgments because of dementia or psychosis. The mental status examination is critical not only for diagnosis but also to provide factual evidence of incompetency.

Index